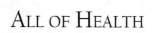

ALL OF HEALTH

ALL OF HEALTH

A Philosophical Dialogue

Nicholas J. Pappas

Algora Publishing
New York

Library of Congress Cataloging-in-Publication Data —

Names: Pappas, Nicholas J., author.
Title: All of health: a philosophical dialogue / Nicholas J. Pappas.
Description: New York: Algora Publishing, [2018] |
Identifiers: LCCN 2018012393 (print) | LCCN 2018014906 (ebook) | ISBN
    9781628943382 (pdf) | ISBN 9781628943368 (soft cover: alk. paper) | ISBN
    9781628943375 (hard cover: alk. paper)
Subjects: LCSH: Well-being—Miscellanea. | Quality of life—Miscellanea. |
    Health—Miscellanea. | Conversation.
Classification: LCC BD435 (ebook) | LCC BD435 .P2684 2018 (print) | DDC
    128—dc23
LC record available at https://lccn.loc.gov/2018012393

Printed in the United States

TABLE OF CONTENTS

Introduction

In this book I present two friends, Director and Physician — a philosopher and, well, a physician. In the course of their larger discussion about health, they arrive at the notion of symbiosis — a living together to the advantage of each.

I do not think it is too much of a stretch to say that a good conversation is sort of living together to the advantage of each. In such conversation, such dialogue, we engage with our hearts and minds. When are we more alive than when so engaged?

What is the peak of health if not this life, this engagement? Director and Physician want to know what health is. But they want more. They want to be healthy. The conversation is not idle. Something vital is at stake. But do they realize that by having their lively conversation about health, they are healthy, if only for a while?

Director and Physician see three basic types of health — bodily, mental, and societal. These three types affect one another. How they affect one another matters, matters in a critical way. Even a friendly conversation about health — perhaps especially such a conversation — can touch on something critical.

But there is more. A friendly conversation allows special access to the critical. Our guard is down in such a conversation. We are less likely to be defensive. We are more likely to keep our minds open and clear. We are likely to feel the confidence it takes to learn.

So remember as you engage with this book — be at ease. Director won't think poorly of you if you laugh at what he says. Physician won't hold a grudge if you don't share his views. Neither of them will mind if you wish

---

1

to pause and consider something more closely, or dismiss something else out of hand.

And I, I only hope one thing — that you will enjoy it. Enjoy the characters, enjoy their interplay; enjoy when they are right, enjoy when they are wrong; enjoy learning something new, enjoy seeing more than the author sees. Above all else enjoy — because, after all, what is health for?

— Nick Pappas

ALL OF HEALTH

Physician: What a wonderful trail! When did you discover it?

Director: I started hiking it when I was a boy. But be careful, Physician. The thaw has made the rocks slippery.

Physician: That's all I need to do is break a leg out here in the middle of nowhere. So how often do you bring friends to hike with you?

Director: On this trail? You're the first.

Physician: Well, I'm honored! But why choose me?

Director: You love to hike. You've been a good doctor to me. And I thought it would be something nice for us to do before you move away across the country.

Physician: Well, I think you're right. It is nice. Very nice. And I'm grateful for the invitation.

Director: You know, we haven't talked much about your move.

Physician: There's not much to say. I'm finally going to teach.

Director: What exactly will you be teaching?

Physician: Health. I'm going to occupy the first endowed chair of health at the university.

Director: Health? As in all of health?

Physician: Yes.

Director: But what an enormous field!

3

Physician: I know it is. But what makes you say so?

Director: For one, there's bodily health. And then there's mental health, assuming you split this off from bodily health. And then there's something we might call societal health.

Physician: Societal health? I hadn't thought of that. But I think you have a point.

Director: How will you teach all of this?

Physician: Well, I won't try to teach it all at once. I'll break it down into manageable pieces. I mean, a history professor doesn't teach all of history at once. A biology professor doesn't try to teach all of biology at once.

Director: True. But they sometimes teach courses explaining what history is, what biology is.

Physician: Introductory courses?

Director: Yes. But the 'what is' question can be the subject of higher level courses, as well.

Physician: So you expect I can teach what health is on all levels.

Director: Of course.

Physician: Maybe I'll save that for later. I want to start with something practical.

Director: Like what?

Physician: Physical fitness.

Director: What do you have to say about that?

Physician: I can talk about exercise. You know, give an overview of all the latest studies on how it affects the body.

Director: Yes, and I suppose you can do the same with diet, and sleep, and so on.

Physician: Of course.

Director: But what about disease?

Physician: What about it?

Director: Doesn't that affect the body?

Physician: Yes, but I think that's a topic for another course.

Director: And in that course you'll teach about contagions and the like?

Physician: Naturally.

Director: But will you teach about other things?

Physician: What other things?

Director: Depression, for one. Is that a disease — or a disorder, or some other sort of thing — that affects the body? Or do you cordon that off as only affecting the mind?

Physician: It can certainly affect the body.

Director: And what about society? Can't a diseased society have an effect on your physical health? Can't it cause stress, and anxiety, and even plain old fear? Those things can't be good for your body, can they?

Physician: Of course not. And they're not good for your mind, either.

Director: Now, your university. Isn't it a sort of society?

Physician: It is.

Director: Is it diseased?

Physician: Well, it's not perfect. But I'm not sure I'd call it sick.

Director: Would you call it a mostly healthy kingdom?

Physician: Kingdom? Ha, ha. I guess it depends who's king.

Director: You are.

Physician: Ha! And why do you say that?

Director: Because your task is the most important on campus.

Physician: Let me guess. The health of my subjects.

Director: That's right. You must teach them health. And they'll learn by making themselves healthy. And you can employ any means you wish toward this end.

Physician: In this, my utopia of health?

Director: I wouldn't call it a utopia. After all, even if you're not king, you'll still speak from a position of authority. So a number of your recommendations might well be adopted in real life.

Physician: Well, I certainly hope they are!

2

Director: Let's hear your definition of health.

Physician: The simple definition is easy. Health is the proper functioning of the body.

Director: Including the body politic?

Physician: Yes, sure. A healthy society is important to our health.

Director: And what about the mind? Or do you say mind is body?

Physician: The mind is body. But the mind is more.

Director: How so?

Physician: There's more to the mind than we know.

Director: There's more to the body than we know.

Physician: True, but the mind is special.

Director: I agree. But how?

Physician: Oh, Director, you of all people should know how.

Director: What if we say this? The mind is special because we can sometimes heal it with words.

Physician: Interesting. I never thought of it that way. But what do we say in order to heal the mind?

Director: We'll have to ask someone who knows, an expert.

Physician: An expert in words?

Director: Yes, but also in manner. Or don't you think that's important?

Physician: Of course I think that's important. But I'm afraid words and manner take us outside the realm of science.

Director: I'm not so sure. But even so, if the words and manner work, why would it matter?

Physician: It matters because we need to know how they work, why they work.

Director: Well, we should make a study. But what if, in the end, we decide it's more a matter of art than science? Would you practice this healing art if you could? Or do you limit yourself to science?

Physician: I'm someone who wants to know reasons.

Director: Then you'll have to explore the more-to-the-mind-than-we-know.

Physician: Agreed.

Director: But do you have any doubt that the more-than-we-know is something physical?

Physician: What else could it be?

Director: I don't know. But if it is physical, does that mean we interact with it in a physical way? So when my mouth speaks healing words, those words touch, physically touch, the other?

Physician: You're saying the words are physical sound waves that travel across the air?

Director: Yes, and then they strike home through the ears to the brain of the other, where they make physical changes.

Physician: That's true, Director. But what's your point?

Director: This might turn out to be more science than art.

Physician: But that's what we want!

Director: So you can teach it from your chair of health?

Physician: Yes!

Director: You really wouldn't teach an art?

Physician: I'll leave that to others. I want to teach what we learn about the more-than-we-know.

Director: That's going to be difficult.

Physician: Oh? Why?

Director: Because it's always difficult to operate along the fringe of the unknown.

Physician: And that's what makes it exciting! Piercing the darkness.

Director: You know, of course, you'll meet resistance if you try to shed light.

Physician: Well, of course. All unknowns resist being known.

Director: Yes, but I'm talking about a different sort of resistance. People will resist you.

Physician: People? Why?

Director: Because many of them consider the 'more-than-we-know' to be the seat of the soul.

3

Physician: But who doesn't want to learn about soul? I think you overstate the resistance.

Director: Maybe. So let's say you figure it out. Will you speak of soul from your chair of health?

Physician: Of course! If we know what soul is, we'll know how to make it well.

Director: So you'll preach the health of the soul?

Physician: Yes, though I don't know that 'preach' is the right word.

Director: What is the right word?

Physician: Teach.

Director: Okay. But I think there's an issue you'll have to face.

Physician: What is it?

Director: Many will say soul is more than mind.

Physician: They'll say our soul is our all?

Director: Yes. So do you know what that means?

Physician: It means people won't believe I have knowledge of soul unless I have knowledge of all.

Director: Are you ready to claim omniscience?

Physician: Ha, ha. Of course not.

Director: But you do want to learn all you can learn about the mind.

Physician: Certainly.

Director: And to the extent the mind is a finite thing, it's possible to learn it all?

Physician: I believe it is.

Director: And if we've learned it all, we can cure all mental illnesses?

Physician: That's the promise.

Director: Is unhappiness a mental illness?

Physician: I would say it is, speaking loosely.

Director: Will you have unhappy students on your campus?

Physician: Almost certainly.

Director: Will you seek them out and try to learn what's wrong?

Physician: Well....

Director: What's the matter? Isn't happiness a matter of health?

Physician: It is.

Director: And you sit the chair of health.

Physician: Director, I can't be responsible for everyone's happiness.

Director: But who says you're responsible? You just want to learn.

Physician: But if I learn I'll want to help.

Director: Then why don't you help?

Physician: Because when will I have the time for all this?

Director: Isn't this just part of your job?

Physician: It's the job of the counselors employed by the school.

Director: Maybe you can teach the counselors what to do.

Physician: Maybe. But counseling doesn't always work.

Director: Why not?

Physician: Sometimes a student won't accept help.

Director: If the school offers help, why would a student refuse?

Physician: Because of pride. Or mistrust.

Director: Or maybe both?

Physician: Yes, maybe both.

Director: What's to mistrust in someone who offers to make you healthy again?

Physician: Yes, but step back a moment. You say 'healthy again'. What if the student was never healthy?

Director: Are you suggesting they might not know what healthy is?

Physician: Yes.

Director: And if they don't know, how can the school?

Physician: That's how the student will likely think.

Director: Who can the student turn to?

Physician: They have to start with themselves.

Director: And what do they do? Say, 'Self, tell me what healthy is'? Maybe they need someone to show them.

Physician: And how will someone do that?

Director: Why, by example.

Physician: So I need to be an example to my students?

Director: That's your responsibility, yes. Do you regret you took the job?

Physician: No, I'm more than ever glad I took it!

Director: Because you know you're the picture of health?

Physician: Because I believe I can do some good.

4

Director: Tell me, Physician. What is mental health?

Physician: It's having a sense of well being.

Director: Everyone who has a sense of well being is mentally healthy?

Physician: Well, I don't know if we can be absolutely strict about it.

Director: Why not?

Physician: Because someone might feel well being at an inappropriate time.

Director: When is it inappropriate to feel well being?

Physician: In the midst of chaos, for instance.

Director: Or while living in a highly dysfunctional world?

Physician: Or that, yes.

Director: And if you feel well being in such a world, you can't be mentally healthy?

Physician: Don't you think that's true?

Director: I don't know. I mean, if you feel good, can the world really be dysfunctional for you? Doesn't it in some way work?

Physician: Yes, but the world isn't made for you alone.

Director: It needs to function for everyone?

Physician: That's the ideal.

Director: Hmm. What if we consider a more narrow example?

Physician: What do you have in mind?

Director: The family. If it works for you, but none of the other members, are you mentally ill?

Physician: Well....

Director: And what if it works for all of the others but not for you?

Physician: You certainly wouldn't have a sense of well being.

Director: Yes. And what if it works for some of the people some of the time, and so on? Don't things get complicated fast?

Physician: Of course.

Director: Then how much more complicated does it get if we talk about society in general?

Physician: It gets very complicated.

Director: So can we ever say society is simply functional or dysfunctional? Or do we have to say functional or dysfunctional for whom and when?

Physician: That would clearly be more accurate.

Director: But not everyone is willing to see it this way.

Physician: How do they see it?

Director: They believe function and dysfunction are absolutes. And this makes them think strange things.

Physician: Such as?

Director: If a social entity functions for them, they think something is wrong with those for whom it doesn't work. Do you know people like this?

Physician: Of course I do. And they often stand in the way of progress.

Director: How do we make progress?

Physician: We change what we can to end the dysfunction.

Director: Then I think we need one important thing.

Physician: What?

Director: Freedom from a sort of illness.

Physician: What illness?

Director: One that makes us have delusions.

Physician: About dysfunction and function?

Director: Yes, delusions that make us mistake the one for the other, and the other way round. Don't you think that happens?

Physician: Yes, that happens.

Director: So what does this mean for you as a teacher?

Physician: I must teach my students to have no delusions. And to have the courage to fix whatever dysfunction they can.

5

Director: Yes, but let's be clear. What is delusion?

Physician: Believing something against all evidence, against all rational argument.

Director: Can you teach students to value evidence, to value rational argument?

Physician: I can try.

Director: Will it help if you tell them delusion can undermine health?

Physician: It might. But what if they're focused on other things?

Director: They don't care about health?

Physician: Sure they do, but what they really care about is happiness. And they see evidence that people can be happy in their delusions, happy in their dreams.

Director: What evidence?

Physician: Radiance among the dreamers.

Director: Radiance? What's that?

Physician: It's an inner glow that shines through.

Director: What causes this glow?

Physician: Belief in a dream.

Director: And what else?

Physician: Well, health.

Director: Which would your students rather have? Health or a dream?

Physician: I think they'd want both.

Director: Why?

Physician: Because health can allow you to pursue your dream. And the dream, if good, can bring you health.

Director: But weren't we equating dreaming with delusion?

Physician: Yes, but now I want to say it's one thing to be a dreamer, and it's another to have a dream.

Director: And by having a dream we mean having a goal.

Physician: Put simply, yes.

Director: And achieving our goal makes us happy?

Physician: Of course.

Director: But if we're dreamers, that can interfere with both health and dream?

Physician: That's certainly true.

Director: Because being a dreamer means you have delusions.

Physician: Right.

Director: What do you have delusions about?

Physician: Often enough? Delusions about yourself.

Director: And how you interact with the world?

Physician: Yes.

Director: But if we're clear about ourselves and the world?

Physician: We have a better chance of achieving both health and dream.

Director: And we need respect for both evidence and rational argument in order to have this better chance?

Physician: Without a doubt.

Director: Do you think the students will see this truth?

Physician: I think they might. But some will want us to strengthen what we're saying.

Director: How so?

Physician: They'll want a guarantee.

Director: What guarantee?

Physician: That freedom from delusion will bring them health, which they can use for their dreams.

Director: But there's more to health than being clear about things. Isn't there?

Physician: Yes, and that's why those who are serious about their dreams will pay close attention in my classes.

Director: Where they'll learn about mental, bodily, and societal health?

Physician: Right, and the need to have all three.

6

Director: Let's set the students aside for now.

Physician: Alright, let's.

Director: Tell me. If your society is sick, can you be well?

Physician: Not completely, at least.

Director: Not even if you have truly amazing personal health?

Physician: You couldn't be fully healthy unless you were somehow stronger than your society.

Director: What does it mean to be stronger than your society? Aren't we all a part of our society?

Physician: Not if we stand apart when it's sick.

Director: Will that be one of the courses you teach, 'Standing Apart'?

Physician: I think it should be, don't you?

Director: What will be on the syllabus?

Physician: I suppose we'll talk about others who stood apart.

Director: And can you know if these others were happy? Or doesn't that matter? Is the fact of standing apart enough?

Physician: When you stand apart from a sick society, happiness will come.

Director: Are you sure? How can you be happy when everyone else is less than well?

Physician: Well, I suppose you have a point.

Director: Maybe you need a band of healthy friends — a society of your own.

Physician: Yes, I think that's an excellent idea. We'll stand together apart.

Director: Should we assume this society will be healthy?

Physician: Yes.

Director: And what about those who make it up? What health is most important to them?

Physician: Mental health is most important here.

Director: And will you ask yourselves what it is, exactly, that makes the larger society sick?

Physician: We'll have to. Asking that is part of mental health. You have to know the reason why you stand apart.

Director: So what could it be?

Physician: Oh, there are many possible reasons.

Director: Name one.

Physician: A collapse in values.

Director: Ah, the most common complaint. Can we raise the values back up?

Physician: I'm afraid when it's gotten to that point, it's too late.

Director: Really? There's no chance of recovering health once lost?

Physician: Not when it's lost like that.

Director: But how can you, a man of healing, think that way?

Physician: I heal things that can be healed. And, accordingly, I know when a body is beyond repair.

Director: And when it's beyond, you let it die?

Physician: Yes, with dignity.

Director: Can society die with dignity?

Physician: Societies, like humans, can die different deaths.

Director: What sort do you prefer?

Physician: The kind where society fades gracefully away.

Director: And then what's left?

Physician: A new one always rises in its place — and starts rising before its death.

Director: And if all of this is gradual enough, is it possible not to notice the change?

Physician: Oh, everyone notices the change — even if we try to smooth things over by calling the new thing by the old name.

7

Director: Can we do that with humans?

Physician: Raise a new one from the old?

Director: Yes, and call it by the same name.

Physician: You'd better give me an example.

Director: Suppose we transplant a heart, or even a brain. Is it the same person?

Physician: Well, with the heart I think it's safe to say it's the same person. But with a brain....

Director: Let's say we keep the same brain. But we transplant every other organ in the body. Is it the same person?

Physician: Yes.

Director: Because the brain is the same?

Physician: Because the brain is the same.

Director: But the brain interacts closely with the rest of the body.

Physician: True.

Director: In changing all the rest of us, our organs, we've changed those interactions.

Physician: Of course.

Director: Doesn't that suggest the brain will have to make some changes, too?

Physician: It no doubt does.

Director: Some serious changes?

Physician: Yes, very serious changes.

Director: But it's still the same person.

Physician: Yes.

Director: Now what about society?

Physician: Well, the organs of a society are its institutions. We can replace those with new ones.

Director: And is the society still the same?

Physician: It depends on the brain.

Director: What's the brain in any society?

Physician: The people.

Director: The people, or the ruling class?

Physician: You have a point. But in a democracy, the people are the ruling class.

Director: And what's the ruling class in, for example, an oligarchy?

Physician: The few.

Director: If we remove the few, the brain, and replace them with a new brain, the many — would it be the same society?

Physician: No, I don't think it would.

Director: Even if we call it by the same name?

Physician: It would be a new society no matter what we say.

Director: Would it be a healthier society?

Physician: Isn't that why we'd make the change?

Director: And healthier societies, they make for healthier members?

Physician: That's the whole point.

Director: Can everyone be made healthier?

Physician: That would be ideal. But no, not everyone benefits from the change.

Director: What happens to those who don't?

Physician: Maybe they go to another society or found a new one of their own.

Director: No two easy things.

Physician: But better than being sick.

Director: True. But what society is willing to take in the sick?

Physician: Well, sick to us might not be sick to them.

Director: I see. But let's say no one wants to take them in. Are they then forced to found a new society of their own?

Physician: If they want to be healthy, yes.

Director: So what's the first thing the new society needs?

Physician: A place to call their own.

Director: Yes, but wouldn't you say the first thing is the people themselves?

Physician: That goes without saying.

Director: Okay. But here's what I wonder. Suppose we're the ones forming the new society, any kind of society. How do we tell who's healthy enough to join? Or do we just let everyone in?

Physician: No, we don't let just anyone in. But to be sure, we're not talking about turning away those with physical ailments.

Director: What kind of ailments concern us? The mental kind?

Physician: Not quite. The moral kind.

Director: The moral isn't mental?

Physician: Why do you ask?

Director: Maybe I should ask what the moral is.

Physician: It has to do with principles of right and wrong.

Director: Where do we hold those principles? In our bodies? In society? Where?

Physician: We hold them in our minds. But let's not get distracted from the point. Someone who, for instance, lies, and cheats, and steals, can't come in.

Director: And what about someone who cheats a little in sports and tells white lies now and then?

Physician: If that's all they do? They're fine with me.

Director: But are you the only one who decides?

Physician: No, of course not.

Director: Who does?

Physician: That's a good question.

Director: Should we establish a council on morality?

Physician: That's a little much, don't you think?

Director: So what do we do?

Physician: I guess we have to make these decisions together.

Director: All of us?

Physician: All those already accepted into our society.

Director: And if we're the first? Who decides on us?

Physician: That's easy, Director. We do.

8

Director: Once we've gathered our members, how do we foster their health?

Physician: We start with their bodies and give them the best physical care.

Director: And their minds?

Physician: We'll have a school where they can learn.

Director: Learn at all ages?

Physician: Yes. But we'll have additional institutions for the young. We'll want to train them.

Director: Train them in what?

Physician: Honesty, reliability, courage.

Director: How do we make sure the training sticks?

Physician: Why wouldn't it?

Director: The young might be exposed to other ways.

Physician: Such as?

Director: The way that praises money.

Physician: Oh, there's nothing wrong with money. In fact, it takes honesty, reliability, and courage to earn it.

Director: It takes courage?

Physician: Sometimes you have to take risks. But look, Director. I understand your concern. We don't want our youths to glorify money. They'll seek it, but only so much.

Director: I'll leave the workings of that to you. But can you imagine other things like this, things like wealth? Things that can be taken too far?

Physician: What have you got in mind?

Director: Power and fame.

Physician: Ah, lust for them has brought many to ruin.

Director: But some say striving for power and fame is good.

Physician: Yes, they say it's good for you and good for society, too.

Director: What do you say to them?

Physician: I tell them moderation is the key.

Director: But can the moderate win even a modest amount of these things against the immoderate?

Physician: Director, what we care about is health, not these things.

Director: Agreed. But how far do you take moderation?

Physician: What do you mean?

Director: Can you be excessive in your moderation?

Physician: I'm not sure I understand.

Director: Can you think of something we shouldn't be moderate in?

Physician: Health. Ha, ha. To be moderate in health is to be excessive in moderation. Now you name something.

Director: Philosophy.

Physician: Ah, I knew you'd say that. So if our society is dedicated to health, what role will philosophy play?

Director: Well, I'm not going to tell you philosophers should rule.

Physician: Ha, ha! Who ever thought they could?

Director: What do you think philosophy is?

Physician: It's clarification. Don't we want things in our society to be as clear as they can be?

Director: Yes, I should hope so. But here's what I think the philosophers will need to clarify — whether health itself can be taken too far.

Physician: Oh, but how can we ever be too healthy? Don't you want perfect health?

Director: But is there a health beyond perfect?

Physician: How could there be?

Director: Look at it this way. What if a perfectly healthy man comes to you and says he wants an operation to enhance the working of his brain. Maybe that's not possible today, but it might be soon, no?

Physician: We're on the cusp of many such things.

Director: Yes. So what will our society do?

Physician: We'll give him the operation.

Director: And do we give it to him for free, or does he have to pay?

Physician: He has to pay.

Director: Do you think everyone would like an operation like this?

Physician: Many, if not all.

Director: But what if not every one of those many can afford the surgery? Do you see what I'm driving at?

Physician: Yes, you're worried about classes forming between the super healthy and the merely healthy.

Director: And that's not even to mention the sick.

Physician: But we can subsidize the poor. So all the sick can become healthy, and the healthy even super healthy one day.

Director: So we've made clear the tendency of our society. Everything will lead toward super health. And the super healthy will strive to become even healthier still. But at a certain point I have to wonder if we're still talking about health.

Physician: What do you mean?

Director: If it's healthy to be able to see something a mile away, is it healthier still to see something ten miles away? Is 'healthier' really the right word? What does health mean?

Physician: It means for things to work well.

Director: Eyes that can see a mile work well. Eyes that can see ten miles work well. Or do you disagree?

Physician: Our definition of working well changes based on what's possible.

Director: So my legs don't work well because someone has legs that move faster than mine?

Physician: I suppose we have to talk about a sort of average. Most people's legs work the way yours work. Some work better, some work worse.

Director: Then is health all about averages?

Physician: That raises an interesting question.

Director: Oh?

Physician: Should medicine aim high or toward the middle?

Director: You mean, aim to make the best legs better still, or aim to bring the bottom half toward the average?

Physician: That's what I'm wondering.

Director: Well, it's our society. How do we want it to be?

Physician: I want it to aim high.

Director: Why?

Physician: Because all boats rise with the tide.

Director: Hmm.

Physician: What is it?

Director: Is that really why? Or is that the justification for what you want?

Physician: And what do I want?

Director: You want the best health you can possibly have.

Physician: Everyone wants that.

Director: Yes, but don't you assume you'll be on top?

Physician: Even so, that doesn't mean the others won't get healthier, too.

Director: That may be true. But if everyone is healthier, and keeps on getting healthier, and no one can make a great leap, aren't we all, for all our progress, essentially, locked into castes?

9

Physician: But why can't people make great leaps?

Director: Well, aside from money, what would it take to make one?

Physician: That's what I'm asking you.

Director: What does it take to recover from a procedure, any sort of procedure? Don't tell me you don't know.

Physician: It takes resilience.

Director: And the greater the procedure, the greater the resilience required?

Physician: Naturally.

Director: What underlies resilience?

Physician: I'm not sure what you have in mind.

Director: Oh, come on, Physician. You act as if you never saw patients recover.

Physician: Alright, it's strength.

Director: Ah, strength.

Physician: Why do you say it like that?

Director: Because I want to know if our society is dedicated to health or strength.

Physician: Don't the two go hand in hand?

Director: Not necessarily. A society can be strong without being healthy, you know.

Physician: What's an example?

Director: Think of certain tyrannies. Aren't their societies sick? And yet these societies are strong enough in some cases to overcome their neighbors. Or is that a bad example?

Physician: No, that's a very good example. But what about the other way round? What good does it do to be healthy but not strong?

Director: Are you worried such a society would be conquered?

Physician: Yes. We have to be able to protect ourselves.

Director: So it's best if strength and health go together.

Physician: Always. Strength belongs to health. And when we say a society is healthy, we imply it's strong. It's unhealthy to be weak.

Director: But unhealthy only because of the threat from others?

Physician: Not necessarily. A weak society can buckle under all on its own.

Director: And what does all this mean for individuals?

Physician: All that it means for societies. And I'll note further that If you're weak, people won't value you as much.

Director: Why not?

Physician: Because strength is always an asset.

Director: But why?

Physician: Director, it's obvious.

Director: Then tell me what's not so obvious.

Physician: People sense that if you're strong, you can offer protection.

Director: But aren't there other ways to protect?

Physician: Name one.

Director: What if, even though you're relatively weak, you help build a protective wall around society? Wouldn't people value and respect you then?

Physician: You have a point.

Director: Yes. And what if you're married to the one who helps build that wall? Respect?

Physician: Maybe. But beyond that it gets ridiculous. What if I'm the pig farmer whose bacon feeds the spouse of the one who builds the wall? Respect?

Director: I, for one, would respect such farmers. Though I'd rather they farmed grain.

10

Physician: Okay, but forget about respect. Let's talk about strength itself.

Director: Alright. Do you want to say strength is always useful in and of itself?

Physician: I do. Though I admit there can be misuse.

Director: I certainly agree. But tell me. Where can we be strong?

Physician: In body or mind.

Director: And sometimes both?

Physician: And sometimes both. And that's what our society will strive to achieve.

Director: Do we always have to strive for strength, or are some of us naturally strong?

Physician: There's definitely a natural strength. But the strength that comes through effort is more important.

Director: Can too much effort be counterproductive?

Physician: What do you mean?

Director: I mean, is it possible to strive so much we make ourselves sick?

Physician: That would take a lot of striving.

Director: Is that rare?

Physician: A lot of striving? It depends on the circles you move in. For some laziness is the norm. For others, well, they strive.

Director: And some of the strivers make themselves sick?

Physician: Yes.

Director: What kind of sickness would it be?

Physician: It depends on what they overdo.

Director: If they overdo it in body?

Physician: They might make themselves sick in body — general exhaustion, for instance.

Director: And if they overdo it in mind?

Physician: They might make themselves sick in mind — a nervous breakdown, for example.

Director: But does it work the other way, too?

Physician: How so?

Director: If I overdo it in mind, might I not make myself sick in body?

Physician: I think that's possible.

Director: And if I overdo it in body, might I not make myself sick in mind?

Physician: You have a point. That might happen.

Director: So any overdoing is bad.

Physician: I completely agree.

Director: Good. But how do we know when we're doing too much?

Physician: That's easy. We'll feel a great deal of pain.

Director: Not the pain of the 'no pain, no gain' variety.

Physician: No, not that. This is something more. Something dangerous.

Director: Now let me ask you this. Is it true that the greater the strength, the further away the pain?

Physician: That's an interesting way to put it.

Director: That's why I put it that way. Is it true?

Physician: Ha, ha. It's true.

Director: Does it hold for society?

Physician: The stronger the society, the further away its pain? Yes.

Director: So does it follow that a strong individual, mentally and physically, in a strong society, will have a long way to go to reach dangerous pain?

Physician: I think it does.

Director: Yes. But here's something that makes me wonder. Aren't there certain pains that don't respect our strength?

Physician: What do you have in mind?

Director: For one, there's the pain of loss.

Physician: That can bring low even the strongest.

Director: When you say 'bring low,' what do you mean?

Physician: In the worst case? The pain triggers serious physical sickness and terrible mental imbalance.

Director: But this doesn't happen to everyone with every loss, at least not to that degree.

Physician: True.

Director: Would it be good to know when someone is susceptible to this?

Physician: So steps can be taken in advance?

Director: Yes.

Physician: It would be good.

Director: How would we know?

Physician: We'd have to perform screenings for something unusual.

Director: Unusual where?

Physician: In the more-than-we-know.

11

Director: You know, if we're going to screen for things, I think we need to make something clear.

Physician: Oh? What?

Director: You can't be expelled for your results.

Physician: Yes, we want to find ways to help people with latent conditions, not drive them out.

Director: And there's another thing we need to make clear. Membership in our society is wholly voluntary.

Physician: Of course it is! You can leave at any time. But who would want to leave?

Director: Those who sense something is wrong.

Physician: Wrong? In what sense?

Director: In the sense that their relationship to our society isn't good.

Physician: You mean our society isn't good for them?

Director: Yes. What do you think?

Physician: It's certainly possible. But will they actually leave?

Director: Why wouldn't they?

Physician: This society might be all they know. And they have connections here.

Director: So it might be hard, but not impossible, to leave for someplace else?

Physician: Yes, hard but not impossible.

Director: Then there's no excuse?

Physician: There's often an excuse for what's hard. But where do you think they'd go? Would you have them found their own society?

Director: Let's say they're attracted to a nearby society, one dedicated to mental health.

Physician: Dedicated purely to mental health? There's no such place.

Director: Why do you say that?

Physician: How would such a society defend itself?

Director: Can we say it has a great enough wall?

Physician: It would be better if it had strong arms.

Director: Then let's say it has strong arms.

Physician: Good. But what if my society, dedicated to bodily strength and the strongest of arms, comes along and attacks your society of mental health?

Director: Oh, it's my society now? Well, we'd have no choice but to use the arms we have, and play mind games on you.

Physician: Ha, ha! And you think you'd succeed?

Director: I think there's a very good chance we would. After all, what controls strength but mind? If we can knock your minds off balance, then bring to bear our not insignificant strength? We might very well win.

Physician: Fair enough. It takes good minds to win at war. Though the healthy have good reason to avoid a fight if they can. Look what's at stake!

Director: Beautiful societies with beautiful members. For health is beautiful, no?

12

Physician: Health is certainly beautiful.

Director: Well, aside from aggressors, what must a beautiful society guard against?

Physician: There are many things. But I would still have it guard against excessive longing for wealth, power, and fame.

Director: What happens if these things aren't pursued in moderation?

Physician: Things get ugly.

Director: Are you sure?

Physician: I have no doubt.

Director: In that case, tell me. What would you do with those who are immoderate?

Physician: After repeated warnings to no avail? I would banish them.

Director: So where would they go? To a society that values immoderation as an engine of excellence, health, and growth?

Physician: I suppose they'd be welcome there.

Director: Yes, and what if they succeed in their new life and gain great influence in that society? Would we have something to fear?

Physician: You mean, the exile might want to take revenge on us?

Director: That's what I mean. What do you think?

Physician: We'd have to be strong enough to ward off attack.

Director: Who would lead our forces? All of us together, or someone in particular?

Physician: We'd need someone in particular.

Director: We'd give this person power, even a very great deal?

Physician: Of course. We'd have to.

Director: And suppose our leader succeeds and we win. Wouldn't he or she deserve fame?

Physician: I suppose.

Director: And what about wealth?

Physician: I have to stop you here. Wealth doesn't necessarily follow from winning the war. Not in an honest society, anyway.

Director: Not even if the leader writes books, gives speeches, consults, and so on?

Physician: Fine, the leader will likely grow rich.

Director: So it's power for at least a time, fame forever — or as 'forever' as forever can be —, and likely riches, too.

Physician: But do you know the important thing?

Director: What is it?

Physician: That these things come from a desire for something else — saving society.

Director: And when we strive to save society, we can do so without moderation?

Physician: Yes, if it's a beautiful society.

Director: You mean if it's one worth saving.

Physician: I do.

Director: So beauty is very important.

Physician: I'm tempted to say nothing is more important.

Director: Yes. But what if someone finds riches, power, and fame to be beautiful?

Physician: They don't belong in our society.

Director: But what if many people find riches, power, and fame to be beautiful? Do we kick them all out?

Physician: I'm not sure we'd kick them all out. But what you're describing is a very great disorder.

Director: What happens with this disorder?

Physician: Many will want to win excessive riches and so on.

Director: And what's the way to win these things in a society like ours?

Physician: Through war.

Director: So what's the temptation?

Physician: To fight many wars.

Director: Aggressive wars?

Physician: Any wars.

Director: Will these wars bring health?

Physician: Defensive wars might. But aggressive wars? Certainly not.

Director: Why are aggressive wars different?

Physician: Because they're unjust!

Director: Even if they serve a beautiful end?

Physician: Ha! What's beautiful in fighting wars for the sake of excess?

13

Director: Then we should say this. 'The beautiful end of war is the defense of a beautiful society.' Yes?

Physician: Yes. But we have to add this. 'Even though war is and will always be ugly.'

Director: Is there anything else we should say?

Physician: No, I think that's it.

Director: And just to be sure, we can be immoderate toward this beautiful end of ugly war?

Physician: If forced to? We can.

Director: Is there a risk our immoderation might make our society sick?

Physician: There certainly is.

Director: What can we do to prevent that from happening?

Physician: Commit ourselves to healing those who show symptoms.

Director: What are the symptoms?

Physician: I can tell you the worst possible symptom. A desire to fight new, aggressive wars.

Director: How do we heal that?

Physician: Honestly? I don't know.

Director: Would you describe this desire as a cancer?

Physician: I think that's a good description, yes.

Director: What do you do with cancer?

Physician: What do you think you do?

Director: You cut it out.

Physician: Yes, but it's not that simple.

Director: You mean, the problem isn't as isolated as it might seem?

Physician: Exactly.

Director: So the sickness spreads in ways we can't always see.

Physician: I think that's true.

Director: And it's not limited to the ones who actually fought.

Physician: No, even those who didn't fight can grow sick.

Director: I wonder. Do you think these problems are peculiar to moderate societies?

Physician: I think that's where they're most pronounced.

Director: Why?

Physician: Because of the contrast.

Director: Between moderation and immoderation.

Physician: Of course.

Director: Does that mean when an immoderate society fights immoderately, everyone simply blends back in at home when the war is over?

Physician: Well, we can't oversimplify things. People always have to adjust after a war, and any adjustment is hard.

Director: But for some it's harder than others? What's hardest?

Physician: Being immoderate in a moderate society.

Director: Because immoderation is the sickness there?

Physician: Yes, and that makes for a very difficult time.

Director: What's the cure?

Physician: For the immoderate to relearn the value of moderation.

Director: And if they don't? Cut the cancer out?

Physician: What does that really mean?

Director: To get rid of the sick.

Physician: In the name of health? Ha!

Director: You don't think it's happened before?

Physician: I'm sure it has.

Director: You know this as a doctor?

Physician: What do you mean?

Director: Have you ever gotten rid of the sick?

Physician: Director, I don't like where you're headed.

Director: I'm headed toward euthanasia.

Physician: Yes, I know. And I know you know that's a completely different thing.

Director: Why?

Physician: Because it involves those who suffer greatly and are terminally ill!

Director: But what about those who are indeed suffering but aren't terminally ill?

Physician: They're just going to suffer and suffer no end?

Director: Yes, what about them?

Physician: They have absolutely no quality of life? No prospect of a cure?

Director: None.

Physician: If they asked me to end their suffering, I would.

Director: What if a small society were sick like this, a society not our own? And they beg, positively beg you to end their suffering.

Physician: They beg for death?

Director: Yes.

Physician: But this is insane. No society is going to ask me this.

Director: Still, what would you do?

Physician: I'd turn to others for advice.

Director: And they say, 'Yes, Physician. Do it. It's only humane.'

Physician: I'd have to know to a certainty there was no chance of a cure for what they were suffering, that they'd just suffer and suffer to no purpose — with zero quality of life.

Director: You said 'to no purpose'. Can suffering have a purpose?

Physician: I think it can.

Director: Can you give an example?

Physician: The suffering might birth valuable insights the sufferer can share.

Director: So the suffering is worth it? Worth enough to keep someone alive despite their wishes?

Physician: We have to help them see the value in life.

Director: You mean, the value of their insights to others.

Physician: Well, yes.

Director: And there can be no other way to get these insights?

Physician: Don't make too much of this. It's just an example.

Director: Okay. But now I'll give an example. Can't we gain insights through suffering the horrors of war?

Physician: The ugly answer to your question is yes.

Director: Do those insights make war worth it? Worth enough not to do away with it if we could?

Physician: I don't know if I'd say that.

Director: Why not?

Physician: Because war is... bad!

Director: Can anything make it less so?

Physician: The only thing that can is justice.

Director: Justice?

Physician: Yes, if justice is served.

Director: Is justice healthy?

Physician: You know it is.

Director: Does that mean the ones with justice on their side are healthier than the others?

Physician: I think there's truth in that.

Director: And they deserve to win?

Physician: Yes.

Director: Now, you're a doctor. Who does a doctor help? The healthy or the sick?

Physician: A doctor helps both, if in different ways.

Director: So you'd help everyone on both sides?

Physician: I'd only help the ones on my side and those we capture.

Director: Why?

Physician: Because we're at war!

Director: Of those on our side and those we capture, who needs the doctor most? The healthy or the sick?

Physician: Obviously the sick.

Director: Are our sick healthier than our sick prisoners?

Physician: Why would they be?

Director: Because our society is healthier than the one we fight.

Physician: Because its cause is more just? I suppose I agree.

14

Director: You've heard of the age of priestesses and priests?

Physician: Of course I have.

Director: What do priestesses and priests do for the ones who fight?

Physician: They often encourage them.

Director: How?

Physician: By telling them their cause is just.

Director: Do both sides have priestesses and priests?

Physician: In one form or another? Yes, of course.

Director: They can be of many and different sorts?

Physician: As many as there are things to believe in, yes.

Director: And it used to be when armies fought, they'd say, 'Our gods are more powerful than theirs'?

Physician: Yes, they certainly would.

Director: And would the most powerful gods always win?

Physician: Well, it's hard to say. If powerful gods can inspire a powerful will in the soldiers, then yes — the most powerful gods will win.

Director: But not if the most powerful gods have three hundred soldiers and the lesser gods have three million.

Physician: In that case, the soldiers of the most powerful gods will put up a terrible, as in awe-inspiring, fight — and lose.

Director: Yes. But tell me, Physician. Are priests and priestesses a mostly healthy lot?

Physician: I suppose it's as it is with anyone. Some are healthy, some are sick.

Director: Do powerful gods speak through the sick?

Physician: I don't know.

Director: So we shouldn't cast out the sickly priests and priestesses?

Physician: No more than we should cast out the rest of the sickly population.

Director: If forced to choose, who should the society save above all others? The healthy or the sick?

Physician: The society should do what I do, and save them all.

Director: And who will do the fighting?

Physician: In war? The healthy, of course.

Director: In other words, the strong?

Physician: Yes.

Director: And what do we do with the strongest of the strong?

Physician: We send them far out front.

Director: Where they can engage the enemy on our own terms?

Physician: Yes, and when we engage on our own terms, we're best suited to survive and conquer. Provided that's the will of the gods.

Director: And what do powerful gods tell us is the aim of health? Being able to fight for them and win?

Physician: What do you think the aim of health is?

Director: To enjoy it.

Physician: Yes, but can't you enjoy a good fight?

Director: Wouldn't you rather enjoy freedom from attack?

Physician: Peace, in other words?

Director: Yes.

Physician: Well, of course, Director. But for most of us, war and peace are out of our control, a matter of chance or fate. So what does it matter what we prefer?

15

Director: I've never known you to sound so helpless.

Physician: That's because no one can overcome luck.

Director: But why worry about that? There are more important things.

Physician: Name one.

Director: Health.

Physician: How can you prove health is more important than luck?

Director: I can ask you this. Which would you rather have? Great health and little luck, or poor health and lots of luck?

Physician: How would you decide?

Director: I'd consider that if my health is poor, I can't enjoy my luck.

Physician: So you'd take great health?

Director: I would. How about you?

Physician: I, too, would take great health. But then we'd both be harried all the time because of our bad luck!

Director: Then let's forget about luck and ask something else. Which would you rather have? Great health or great insight?

Physician: Let me clear up the question. It's great health and poor insight, or poor health and great insight?

Director: Yes.

Physician: But is that really how it goes? Why wouldn't the healthy have great insight?

Director: I'm starting to think I asked a bad question.

Physician: Maybe you did. But let's see where it leads. Let's make the case for great insight coming from poor health.

Director: Alright. Then I think we should start here. Do the healthy pay much attention to the sick?

Physician: Do they pay attention, for instance, to the poor, sick, homeless man on the street? For the most part? Not really.

Director: And what about the sick? Do they pay attention to the healthy?

Physician: I think they do. They study the healthy very closely.

Director: Why?

Physician: They either admire, envy, or despise their health.

Director: So the sick aren't all that interesting to the healthy, but the healthy are very interesting to the sick?

Physician: Yes. But we have to note that there are many healthy people who take great interest in the sick. There are professionals like me. And there are charities, and volunteers, and so on. And that says nothing of those with loved ones who are sick.

Director: Now what about insight?

Physician: The sick have the advantage.

Director: Why? How do we gain insight?

Physician: By making a very close study.

Director: And no one studies like the sick? You're healthy. Do you study your sick patients?

Physician: Well, yes, of course.

Director: Do you gain insights from them?

Physician: I do.

Director: So you have health and insight both.

Physician: Yes, but it's best to have insight into both sick and healthy alike.

Director: Who has that?

Physician: I like to think I do, for one.

Director: How do you have insight into the healthy?

Physician: When you work with the sick, you come to see things about the healthy that even they themselves don't see.

Director: You mean, for instance, what they take for granted?

Physician: Yes, and what they ignore.

Director: Would someone once healthy, who grew sick, but then grew well again, have similar insight?

Physician: You know, they might even have greater insight, assuming they were truly sick.

Director: How sick would they have to be?

Physician: Sick enough that recovery was in doubt.

Director: Would such a person make a good leader?

Physician: If they have leadership skills? Yes, of course. We want our leaders to have great insight.

Director: What else do we want them to have?

Physician: Perspective, and a sense of what's truly important in life.

Director: We want them to have true vision.

Physician: Yes, which they can achieve through surviving the sickness and making their recovery.

Director: But there's a risk.

Physician: The risk they won't get well?

Director: Yes, but I'm thinking of something else. Isn't there a danger the sickness will leave them embittered?

Physician: How so?

Director: Do you agree the kind of illness we're talking about can turn your world upside down?

Physician: Yes, of course I agree.

Director: And if it does, you have to right things somehow?

Physician: Yes.

Director: Righting takes a great deal of effort, no?

Physician: There's no doubt about that.

Director: And not everyone makes this effort?

Physician: You're talking about the healthy? Well, it's true. Not all of the healthy have their worlds turned upside down.

Director: If you were making a terrible effort to turn things right side up, might you not resent those who didn't need to make such an effort?

Physician: I wouldn't. But I take your point. There are those who would.

Director: Do you think it's possible for these people to base their world view on their resentment?

Physician: It's possible. And it's an awful thing.

Director: Why, exactly?

Physician: Why? Because they ruin their vision!

Director: Would we want them to lead?

Physician: Ha! Certainly not.

Director: How do we ensure someone like this never becomes a leader?

Physician: We need a reliable way to screen.

Director: We're looking for true vision, true perspective?

Physician: Yes, but now that you mention it — how do we know what that perspective is?

Director: We have to have it ourselves.

Physician: But then why don't we ourselves lead?

Director: Because perspective alone isn't enough. It takes leadership traits, as you mentioned — the most important of which is being able to act on what you see. Not all of us can.

Physician: Oh, I don't know about that. If you can see, you can do — do something, at least. That's what I believe.

16

Director: Tell me, Physician. Have we been speaking only of physical illness, or did we mean mental illness, as well?

Physician: We meant all illness. But what mental illness do you have in mind?

Director: Hubris.

Physician: A lot of people would say that's not a mental illness, Director.

Director: But it's a bad way of being in the mind, no?

Physician: It is.

Director: Can those with hubris attain to true vision?

Physician: If they're cured? I suppose.

Director: But if they're not?

Physician: They'll be too wrapped up in their excessive pride.

Director: What about those with depression?

Physician: Can they have true vision? Well, are they cured?

Director: No, let's say they're not.

Physician: Depending on how bad it is, I think they can reach true vision.

Director: Hubris must be cured but depression not? Why?

Physician: Because depression and hubris are very different things.

Director: How so?

Physician: Oh, you know how so. Haven't you heard of being blinded by pride?

Director: I have. But can't we be blinded by depression?

Physician: There have been studies showing depressed people have more realistic views on certain things than those who are happy.

Director: I don't doubt they do. But are those with hubris happy?

Physician: I think it depends on whether they meet with success.

Director: Who would give them success?

Physician: Society.

Director: Why would society do that?

Physician: Because society tends to reward those who believe in themselves and execute on that belief.

Director: But won't the hubris grow with the reward?

Physician: Yes, and here's what's worse. Society believes in the success it confers.

Director: What does that mean?

Physician: It means hubris is overlooked or forgiven.

Director: Hmm.

Physician: What are you thinking?

Director: Is it the belief in yourself that's bad?

Physician: For hubris? No, of course not. It's good to believe in yourself.

Director: But you shouldn't believe too much?

Physician: I wouldn't say that. Complete belief in yourself can be very good.

Director: Then what makes hubris bad?

Physician: The pride.

Director: Pride is different than belief?

Physician: Yes, of course. You can't have too much belief. But you can, without a doubt, have too much pride.

Director: How do you know how much is too much?

Physician: Well, it's an art, not a science.

Director: But are there any guidelines to follow?

Physician: Let me give you a clear example that can serve as one. You sacrifice troops on the field of battle solely to secure your pride as a leader.

Director: And that's too much pride.

Physician: Yes, and blindness, too. But there's more we can say.

Director: Oh?

Physician: You're more than sick with pride. You're a monster for acting this way.

Director: Can we define 'monster' as having pride that's out of control?

Physician: Out of control, yes. That's a fine definition.

Director: How do we control our pride?

Physician: We, the healthy? We only take it up to a point.

Director: So monsters either don't know what that point is, or they do and they don't care?

Physician: Exactly. And then society must step in.

Director: What can it do?

Physician: First it must try praise and blame, to encourage good behavior and discourage the bad.

Director: And when that doesn't work?

Physician: Then it employs stronger means.

17

Director: Can it ever be healthy to have boundless pride?

Physician: Never.

Director: Then all the healthy have their pride under control?

Physician: Yes, of course.

Director: But do we all have the potential to lose control?

Physician: That's a good point. I think we do.

Director: If that's true, then isn't having a healthy society more important than ever?

Physician: Yes, because society picks up where we ourselves fail.

Director: But is that all a healthy society is? A means of reining us in?

Physician: No, of course not. But what do you think a healthy society is?

Director: I think it's a big question. But we can start by saying a healthy society is one in which everyone has their place.

Physician: A good place?

Director: If a place is yours, isn't it by definition good?

Physician: If it's truly yours, I'd have to agree.

Director: How can you tell a place is truly your own?

Physician: It just fits.

Director: You mean it's comfortable?

Physician: Yes.

Director: So comfort is the key to health?

Physician: Comfort is part. But it's the sense of belonging that really brings health.

Director: Health for both the individual and society?

Physician: Well, if enough individuals are in a good place, are healthy, won't society, too, have health? Isn't that how you define it?

Director: Yes, but now I'm wondering. Say we have a society of two healthy people.

Physician: You can have a society with only two people?

Director: That's how it seems to me. So if we have this healthy society, and a third comes along looking for a place, but there isn't one with a true fit — what do we do?

Physician: Is it a pretty good fit?

Director: It's pretty good.

Physician: Then we might let them stay.

Director: Is the society now less healthy than it was?

Physician: I suppose it is.

Director: Does it work in the opposite way as well?

Physician: You mean, two people with less than good fits invite a third to join them who has a very good fit?

Director: Yes. Is the society now healthier than it was?

Physician: It is — unless the third one grows sick from constant contact with the other two. But all this gets very complicated as society grows. So let's not get tangled up here.

Director: Okay. But what more can we say about the health of society?

Physician: When society gets large enough, it needs to establish institutions that favor health.

Director: Can you give an example of how an institution might favor health?

Physician: Sure. It might regulate work. It might ensure no one works too much.

Director: Well, then it will need a way of dealing with supply and demand.

18

Physician: How so?

Director: Suppose you're a tailor. You make clothing fit. But there's only one of you and a great many customers. You can't keep up with demand.

Physician: So either I work myself sick and meet the demand, or some people go around with ill fitting clothes.

Director: Yes. And there's more. Are ill fitting clothes good for mental health?

Physician: They certainly don't help.

Director: So how do you keep your health while supporting the health of others?

Physician: I take on apprentices, people I'll train in the trade. More supply to meet the demand.

Director: And when the demand is met?

Physician: Everyone's clothing fits.

Director: But when the clothing all fits?

Physician: There will be less demand.

Director: And what of the apprentices then?

Physician: I'll have to let some of them go.

Director: They'll go off on their own and compete with you?

Physician: I suppose they will.

Director: Is that what you'd call healthy competition?

Physician: Not if they drive me out of business.

Director: But if you drive them out of business?

Physician: That's healthier for me.

Director: Really? You wouldn't feel bad?

Physician: I'd feel worse if I couldn't support myself.

Director: So you'd just accept that some of your former apprentices might be out of luck?

Physician: I'd have to. And I know what you'll say. Our society loses some health, because not everyone has a place.

Director: Would it be better if society made you all have a place?

Physician: Employment for every tailor in the land?

Director: Yes.

Physician: Despite less demand?

Director: Despite less demand.

Physician: But then there's too much supply.

Director: What does that mean?

Physician: Less work for me.

Director: Do you mind working less?

Physician: I mind having less profit.

Director: Why?

Physician: Because I want certain things.

Director: Gold watches and the like?

Physician: Oh, not gold. But would I like to afford a decent watch? Sure.

Director: Does your decent watch bring health?

Physician: It might bring a bit of mental health.

Director: In the form of self-esteem?

Physician: Yes. It's nice to have a nice watch.

Director: I agree. But what if there aren't enough watches to go round, not enough to make for self-esteem?

Physician: You're really talking about nice things in general, not just watches?

Director: Yes. How many nice things does a society need?

Physician: Oh, Director. We don't really need nice things for self-esteem.

Director: What do we need?

Physician: We need to belong.

Director: What happens to those who don't belong?

Physician: For the most part? They grow unhealthy.

Director: Then it seems we've found your place.

Physician: What do you mean?

Director: You'll serve the unhealthy who don't belong. Because physicians heal the sick.

19

Physician: But what if the situation is hopeless?

Director: Would you really see it that way?

Physician: Why, do you think I always have hope?

Director: I think you think hope always does good.

Physician: Well, if someone is hopeless, and I give them hope, won't that make them stronger?

Director: It very well may. But isn't there a negative alternative?

Physician: What alternative?

Director: The one that comes when the hope proves false. What happens then?

Physician: They sink into depression.

Director: So you recognize that hope has a bearing on health.

Physician: Of course I do. When it comes to mental health, hope is the one true cure. And hope even helps with physical health. It can chase certain ailments away, or make you feel them less.

Director: And what about society? Does hope help there?

Physician: It does. Exactly in the same way.

Director: Hope can burn up any malaise? It can fill society with vigor?

Physician: Yes.

Director: But if the hope proves false?

Physician: It's as it is with individuals.

Director: Who can give a society hope?

Physician: A leader.

Director: An elected leader?

Physician: Any sort of leader.

Director: Does the leader share the hope he or she gives to the hopeless?

Physician: Not necessarily.

Director: Oh?

Physician: This person can lack such hope — and that can be an advantage.

Director: An advantage? Tell me how so.

Physician: Hope carries us. But we don't want our hope giver to be carried away.

Director: You don't think there's something cynical in this?

Physician: Cynical? There's something practical in it.

Director: But things are bleak without hope. Or aren't they?

Physician: I'm not saying the leader has no hope. I'm saying it's hope in something else.

Director: Can you say what it is?

Physician: It's hard to say.

Director: Okay. But what hope in particular does the leader give?

Physician: Hope for a healthy place, one that's a natural fit.

Director: How can anyone promise such a good fit?

Physician: By knowing they have the right tailors.

Director: That sounds very good. But who pays the bill?

Physician: We all do.

Director: Even those who are already happy in their place?

Physician: Yes.

Director: Do you really think we can persuade them to pay? What do you think they'll say?

Physician: Oh, I know what many will say. 'Things have gone fine up to this point. And they'll continue so, as long as we make no changes.'

Director: So their hopes differ from the hopes of those without a good place.

Physician: In many respects? Yes, of course.

Director: Then it's hope against hope?

Physician: It is. But only until we turn all the hopes — to point in the same direction.

20

Director: And how will that happen?

Physician: Through having a common cause.

Director: A typical common cause is war. Is that what you recommend?

Physician: No, there are other causes.

Director: Such as?

Physician: Increasing economic output.

Director: Hmm. Yes. But what else?

Physician: Do you want to hear what the best cause is?

Director: Of course.

Physician: Loving each other.

Director: Love is a cause?

Physician: Love is a cause.

Director: And love gives us hope?

Physician: Love gives us hope. And I know from experience, love makes us well.

Director: Is it the love that makes us well, or is it the hope?

Physician: It's both.

Director: So society should employ them both?

Physician: Well....

Director: What is it?

Physician: I'm fine with society giving us hope. But when it comes to love....

Director: What's different about love?

Physician: There's nothing more personal. So do we really want society to 'employ' it toward however good an end?

Director: I think I see what you're saying. Love should never be a means. Love is an end. But what about hope? How does society give us that?

Physician: Society, through its leader, promises us a place, as we said.

Director: 'Place' in an expansive sense.

Physician: Yes, but also narrowly speaking.

Director: So if I'm a skilled mechanic, society might give me a place in a good shop?

Physician: The shop would give you that place.

Director: Yes, but isn't the shop part of society?

Physician: Of course. But you said the shop is good. What do you mean by that?

Director: What do you think I mean?

Physician: You could mean the shop puts out good work.

Director: And what's wrong with that?

Physician: Nothing. Unless the workers are unhappy.

Director: Why would they be unhappy?

Physician: Because the boss is a tyrant.

Director: So the boss is unhappy, too?

Physician: It's funny you should ask. Yes, tyrants aren't happy.

Director: Are tyrants without hope?

Physician: They are.

Director: Do you think we should have a hopeless tyrant at the head of our society?

Physician: Of course not.

Director: But we can have leaders who have no hope?

Physician: No. The leaders have hope. But, as I said, it can be a different hope.

Director: What is this hope? The hope that all their followers will come to have hope?

Physician: You've described it perfectly! And you know what they say?

Director: Hope begets hope.

Physician: Yes.

Director: But in order for this to work, there's one iron condition.

Physician: And what's that?

Director: That all this hope is grounded... in what's real.

21

Physician: But what's real? The possible or the likely?

Director: That's a good question. How many people do you think put their hopes in something that's possible but very unlikely?

Physician: I think many people do.

Director: Are they happy?

Physician: When what they hope for doesn't come to be? Of course not.

Director: But if they put their hopes into something likely?

Physician: They're more likely to be happy.

Director: Is health very unlikely?

Physician: Health? I think it all depends.

Director: So it's possible for health to be likely?

Physician: Yes.

Director: And if it's likely, what does it take to achieve it? Grounding in what's real, or flight into fancy?

Physician: Grounding in what's real.

Director: Now, part of that is knowing what it means to be healthy.

Physician: Obviously.

Director: What does it mean to be healthy?

Physician: To be healthy is to thrive.

Director: And if I ask what it means to thrive? Will you tell me it means to be healthy?

Physician: It means to allow your personality to develop to its fullest.

Director: I take it you're speaking of those with good personalities.

Physician: Naturally.

Director: How do we know a personality is good?

Physician: How do we know anything is good?

Director: I suppose we'd say it's good for us. So can others' personalities be good for us, or are they only good for them?

Physician: They can be good for both. And that's what a good personality is.

Director: You have a good personality, Physician. And I know it's good for me.

Physician: You, too, have a good personality, Director. And you're a good friend to me.

Director: So we both thrive in our friendship?

Physician: Yes.

Director: Which means we're healthy.

Physician: Of course.

Director: But if we weren't healthy, we wouldn't thrive, which means we wouldn't develop our good personalities to the fullest, which means our friendship would suffer. Yes?

Physician: I think it's true.

Director: And let's make something clear. Can your good personality withstand an illness?

Physician: You mean like coming down with the flu? Certainly.

Director: What about a chronic illness?

Physician: Even with a chronic illness your good personality can remain.

Director: So we're saying we can thrive while sick?

Physician: It's not easy, but it's possible, yes.

Director: And does it make it any easier if our society is sick?

Physician: No, not at all.

Director: Society has a bearing on our health.

Physician: There's no doubt about that.

Director: And therefore a bearing on our friendship?

Physician: That's a hard question, you know.

Director: Why?

Physician: Who likes to think their friendship would be affected by something so far out of their control?

Director: Yes, but it's still best to live in a healthy society. Isn't it?

Physician: Of course it is. But I want to note that it's possible to be very good friends in a society that's sick. So what do you think that means for all we've said?

Director: That's something we might explore. But right now I wonder if you think a healthy society can make someone sick.

Physician: Why would it?

Director: Maybe it's not that person's kind of society.

Physician: Didn't we talk about this? We said that person can leave. But we didn't discuss the other alternative.

Director: Which is?

Physician: That person can change their life.

Director: Change to fit in well?

Physician: That's right.

Director: But what about the other way round?

Physician: Change the society to make it fit you? But you said the society is healthy!

Director: Maybe it's not healthy enough.

Physician: So what can we do?

Director: Before we do anything, it helps to know if we're at the tipping point.

Physician: What do you mean?

Director: Society might be ready for a change and all it takes is one little push.

Physician: Somehow I don't think it's ever that simple.

Director: Let's look at an example. Suppose there are one hundred people in a society. And ten of them are superbly healthy and happy — so much so that the society enjoys a terrific reputation.

Physician: That's fine. But what about the other ninety?

Director: Them? Oh, they're miserable and sick.

Physician: And all of this is because of the way the society is?

Director: Yes, let's say it is.

Physician: Then that society has reached the point.

Director: Has it? Why?

Physician: Oh, you know why. There's too great a disparity.

Director: The ninety will push to tip society into something new? Something that suits them better?

Physician: Certainly.

Director: Is it certain? But what about the ten?

Physician: They'll feel what it's like to be the way the ninety were.

Director: I think that's a mistake.

Physician: Oh? How should things be?

Director: We want everyone to be healthy and happy. Don't we?

Physician: That would be ideal, Director. But things never work that way.

22

Director: Not even in a very small society?

Physician: How small?

Director: Almost as small as can be — the two of us and an imagined third.

Physician: And we're looking for the health and happiness of each to be equal and much?

Director: That's the goal. Now, suppose we're doing fine, and we're nearly equal in happiness and health. But then our third falls sick.

Physician: And that means no more equality?

Director: Yes. Is there anything we can do?

Physician: We can nurse our friend back to health.

Director: Would that negatively affect our happiness or health?

Physician: Why, no. Caring for our sick friend would make us feel good.

Director: And if good, then happy and healthy?

Physician: Very much so.

Director: And what about our friend?

Physician: Even if we can't make them completely whole, they'll be happy to see we care.

Director: What happens in a larger, unhealthy society?

Physician: I'm not sure what you're after.

Director: Isn't there more need to help others there?

Physician: Almost certainly. The society affects their health.

Director: So we can be more happy and healthy in that place?

Physician: What do you mean? I don't see how we could.

Director: There would be more sick people to care for. And caring for people makes us feel good.

Physician: Ha, ha. I wouldn't say that without qualification.

Director: Is it only in caring for our friends that we feel good?

Physician: It's complicated, Director.

Director: And that's why it's best to keep societies small?

Physician: Even small societies can be sick.

Director: So what can we do?

Physician: We can be strong.

Director: Is it true that the stronger we are the more care we can give?

Physician: Yes, of course.

Director: And the stronger we are, the more potential we have for health?

Physician: I think that's true.

Director: Health in what?

Physician: Body and mind.

Director: What if we're healthy only in body?

Physician: And sick in mind and society? Then bodily health amounts to nothing.

Director: Why?

Physician: Because mental and societal sickness will undermine bodily health.

Director: Just as bodily and societal sickness will undermine mental health?

Physician: Not necessarily.

Director: What? Mind on its own can overcome bodily and societal sickness?

Physician: You know full well it can.

Director: Tell me how we know this is so.

Physician: From the example of certain great minds.

Director: I can imagine how a great mind can overcome a sickly body. But how can a great mind overcome a sickly society?

Physician: By telling it how much better it can be.

Director: That's all it takes?

Physician: That's no small thing!

Director: Does this involve telling society how sick it actually is?

Physician: Yes.

Director: What happens when a healthy mind tells a sick society truth?

Physician: Usually? Nothing good. At least for a generation or two.

Director: This mind must expect no success in its own time?

Physician: Don't you think that's true?

Director: I don't know. I'm inclined to think something good can happen right away.

Physician: But how? A sick society never listens at first to what a great mind says.

Director: Yes, but there's society — and then there are individuals.

Physician: Well, of course — the truth might help heal an individual here and there.

Director: Can those individuals help heal society?

Physician: They can make a start. It's an enormous task, you know.

Director: I do. And we can't be intimidated by it.

23

Physician: I think healers need to concentrate their efforts.

Director: How can they best do that?

Physician: By focusing on mental health.

Director: And what comes next after mental health?

Physician: Bodily health, followed by societal health.

Director: But shouldn't societal health be second? After all, an unhealthy society stands a good chance of undermining our mental health. We're not all great minds, you know.

Physician: True. But I'd like to hear more about why you think society has that power.

Director: Society touches us in just about every possible way.

Physician: How so?

Director: To answer that we have to ask what society is.

Physician: It's how we live together.

Director: If we don't live well together, how will we feel?

Physician: We'll feel awful.

Director: And if we feel awful for a long enough period of time?

Physician: We'll likely grow sick.

Director: Mentally sick or physically sick?

Physician: Maybe both.

Director: Then how can we put societal health in last place?

Physician: I guess we can't.

Director: So what's our order of treatment?

Physician: Mental, societal, physical.

Director: Is that the order you'd follow in your own case?

Physician: I think I'd start with societal health.

Director: Why?

Physician: Because I'm already healthy in body and mind.

Director: You're a healthy individual.

Physician: Yes. And when I turn to society I do so for the sake of the individual.

Director: Because society exists for the sake of individuals and not the other way round?

Physician: Just so.

Director: And it's in the interest of society for its individuals to be healthy.

Physician: Of course.

Director: So it should take care of them all, no matter if they're healthy or sick?

Physician: Without a doubt.

Director: And when it takes care, where should it focus?

Physician: On mental health.

Director: How can it tell someone is mentally ill?

Physician: It's often obvious.

Director: How so?

Physician: There might be hallucinations, psychosis, severe depression.

Director: Are there other signs?

Physician: Yes, but this seems a good place to start.

Director: Of the three, psychosis interests me most. Would you mind saying what it is?

Physician: It's a disorder in which thought and emotions are so impaired that contact with external reality is lost.

Director: Can we take this in a loose sense?

Physician: Of course. We can take anything we've been saying in a loose sense.

Director: So, loosely speaking, who tends to become psychotic?

Physician: Ha, ha. I'll tell you who. Authoritarian leaders.

Director: Because they lose touch?

Physician: Yes.

Director: What happens to society under such a leader?

Physician: It might very well become sick.

Director: Society might lose touch?

Physician: It's possible.

Director: Similarly, if such a leader suffers from hallucinations, society might come to hallucinate?

Physician: Sure.

Director: What can the healthy do?

Physician: They can work for society's health.

Director: And?

Physician: And what?

Director: You know what.

Physician: Ha! The healthy must drive the leader from power.

24

Director: Let's forget about sick leaders for now. I want to talk about individuals.

Physician: What kind of individuals?

Director: Sick individuals. What are the ways to cure them?

Physician: Well, we just mentioned truth. And I think there's truth in medicine and therapy.

Director: I see how there can be truth in therapy. But in medicine?

Physician: There's truth when drug and biology match.

Director: Does that depend on society?

Physician: What? Of course not.

Director: But therapy depends?

Physician: In what sense?

Director: It has to take society into account. Or does therapy take place in a vacuum?

Physician: No, it takes society into account.

Director: What do therapists do when society is sick?

Physician: They take it on.

Director: Does that make them subversive?

Physician: Subversive for health? Ha, ha. Yes.

Director: Will society frown on those they heal?

Physician: That's a good question. I don't know.

Director: If it does, would people rather be sick and avoid the frowns?

Physician: I know some who would.

Director: How does this apply to society?

Physician: Is a sick society afraid of frowns? Yes, and so it lashes out against those who do.

Director: Why is it so afraid?

Physician: It desperately needs the approval of others.

Director: Why?

Physician: Ha, ha. The concept is alien to you, I see.

Director: Do you need the approval of others?

Physician: Others I admire, yes.

Director: And if you don't get that approval, do you lash out?

Physician: Of course not.

Director: Why not?

Physician: Because I know that when they don't approve, I'm probably doing something wrong.

Director: Maybe you are. But can't a sick society think that way?

Physician: Think like me? No. But a mostly healthy society might.

Director: It would think it's likely doing something wrong and seek to change its ways?

Physician: Yes, just as you or I would seek to change.

Director: But what if we know we shouldn't change? What if we know the ones we admire just can't see our good for what it is?

Physician: Then why would we admire them?

Director: Hmm. I think you're on to something important.

Physician: How so?

Director: Can we only admire people or societies that see us for what we are?

Physician: I think that's a good rule of thumb.

Director: Yes, and isn't it easy for our society to see us for what we are?

Physician: Why would you say that?

Directory: Because our society helps shape what we become.

Physician: True.

Director: And if it shapes us well, if we become healthy — won't we admire it?

Physician: Of course. But while it's true society might do some of the basic shaping, we do the rest, which is the bulk of it.

Director: But aren't there those who simply let themselves be shaped, almost completely shaped?

Physician: Yes, there are. But let me ask you this. We know if we let a sick society shape us completely, we'll be sick. Do you agree?

Director: Yes.

Physician: Well, what if we let a healthy society shape us completely? Will we be healthy?

Director: I think it depends.

Physician: On what?

Director: How much value we place on being an individual.

Physician: Ah, that's an excellent point. If we want some individual control over our lives, and we don't get it, how can we be healthy?

Director: Yes. But let's put the extreme case. Total health and no control, or total control and no health. Which would you choose?

Physician: I honestly don't know. Who wouldn't want total health? But who wants no control?

Director: Oh, I think there are plenty of people who would take no control. They'd probably describe their situation as liberating.

Physician: You may have a point.

Director: And I suspect there are those who would take total control — because, well, they love control.

Physician: Okay. But these extremes really are a bit too much. Aren't things always something of a mix?

Director: That might be true. But we still have to decide what goes into the mix. So which do you like better? Health or control?

Physician: If I'm in control, you can bet there will be health.

Director: How can you be so sure?

Physician: Because I truly value health.

Director: Mental health?

Physician: All of health.

Director: But is there anything you'd single out as important?

Physician: Sure, the lack of psychosis.

Director: Why that?

Physician: Because, speaking loosely, it's important to keep in touch with external reality.

Director: Is that your definition of mental health? Keeping in touch?

Physician: There's more to it than that.

Director: You mean, you might be in very good touch with external reality and it depresses you?

Physician: Sure, but then you have to try your best to change that reality, to whatever degree you can.

25

Director: Should we say something about hallucinations?

Physician: Sure. Individual or societal?

Director: Societal. But first, what's a hallucination?

Physician: The apparent perception of something not present.

Director: So if a sick society believes it perceives lots of health, it's hallucinating?

Physician: Ha, ha. It is.

Director: And if a sick society believes it perceives enemies everywhere?

Physician: And those enemies really aren't there? Hallucination, or rather, paranoia.

Director: Now, the cure must be to get society to stop thinking its seeing what's not there. Yes?

Physician: Yes.

Director: How do we do that?

Physician: We have to prove it's not there.

Director: Is that an easy thing to do?

Physician: Proving a negative? To a sick society? No, it's very hard.

Director: What do we have to do?

Physician: We must bear witness to the truth.

Director: And if society pays us no mind?

Physician: We still serve as examples.

Director: Why?

Physician: Because there will always be those who believe us.

Director: Believe our negative truth.

Physician: Yes.

Director: How far should we be willing to go for this truth?

Physician: As far as health allows.

Director: Then there's no sacrifice involved?

Physician: Oh, there's sacrifice. You can sacrifice time, money, your career, relations with others.

Director: But do some ever go too far and sacrifice their health?

Physician: Yes, that happens.

Director: What's that like?

Physician: What's it like? It's tragic.

Director: Do you think people enjoy tragedy?

Physician: The majority of people enjoy tragedy when it's not their own.

Director: But they don't like to admit it?

Physician: Who likes to admit a weakness for that?

Director: But that's odd, isn't it?

Physician: Why is it odd?

Director: Because they can afford to admit the weakness.

Physician: Because they're the majority?

Director: Yes. Don't you think the majority is always strong?

Physician: No, I don't. The majority can be strong. But it can also be weak.

Director: When is it weak? When indulging in tragedy?

Physician: It's weak when it's delusional.

Director: Hmm. And would you say that's how it is with any ruling power?

Physician: You're wondering if, for instance, a delusional king is weak?

Director: I am. I mean, doesn't the delusional king still have the power of a king?

Physician: The king's power will waste away as it's used to no good end.

Director: Really? Then maybe the king needs some help.

Physician: What do you have in mind?

Director: Could you, as physician to the king, help him put his power to good use?

Physician: Well, if I won some influence with him....

Director: So you would serve a sick king?

Physician: It depends on how sick.

Director: If only a little sick?

Physician: I'd serve.

Director: But massively sick?

Physician: A greatly delusional king? I don't like to back down from a challenge. But I'm not sure what good I could do.

Director: Then what's to be done? Will the realm simply have to suffer with no hope of its king getting well?

Physician: You're appealing to the martyr in me, you know.

Director: Yes, but what if you're clever?

Physician: How so?

Director: You show him one thing about external reality at a time.

Physician: And we just build our way up?

Director: Is there any other way?

Physician: It depends how strong he is.

Director: What do you mean? Isn't a delusional king weak?

Physician: Yes, but there can be inner strength, beyond the delusion.

Director: So what would you do?

Physician: I might decide to shock him with all the truth at once. If he's weak, it'll be too much, and he might have a sort of collapse. But if he's strong? The shock might wake him up.

Director: But if he's neither weak nor strong but something in between?

Physician: Then he might turn on me — and make my life hell.

26

Director: So much for kings. But do these things hold for a people, too, a greatly delusional people?

Physician: I don't see why they wouldn't. Delusion is delusion.

Director: So the people might have a sort of collapse if you show them all the truth at once?

Physician: If they're weak in their inner selves? Yes. Don't you agree?

Director: I don't know. I think before they'd collapse they simply wouldn't believe you.

Physician: And if they're a strong people?

Director: Then they definitely wouldn't believe you.

Physician: Oh, come on. If they're truly strong, there's a good chance they'll wake up.

Director: Okay. But I think we usually have something of a mix.

Physician: The people are strong and weak at once?

Director: Yes. Some are strong enough for truth. Others aren't.

Physician: Then the people as a whole might be in-between. And like the in-between king....

Director: So what's the solution?

Physician: It's as you said. We have to be clever. We offer up a single truth.

Director: And when the delusional people have digested that?

Physician: We give them another. And so on.

Director: But here's something I wonder. How will you feed the strong and weak? Don't they digest at different rates?

Physician: Well, that's true. It's a problem.

Director: Yes. And isn't it aggravated if society is divided up into strong and weak, with nothing in between?

Physician: Of course it is.

Director: Can such a society ever be whole?

Physician: Well, the parts make up the whole, even though they're unlike.

Director: What if part of a part breaks away? Is society less than whole?

Physician: Maybe for a time. But it'll have to adjust.

Director: Would it be easier for society to try to stop these people from breaking away?

Physician: It depends.

Director: On what?

Physician: On whether the society is more healthy or sick.

Director: What if it's more healthy?

Physician: It's easier to let them go.

Director: Really? Why?

Physician: Because healthy societies adjust, or heal, more quickly.

Director: And if the society is more sick?

Physician: It's easier to force those who would leave to stay.

Director: Alright. But we've been considering people who want to leave. Does a society ever tell people to go?

Physician: An unhealthy society might.

Director: Only an unhealthy society? I feel like we're forgetting something here. But who would an unhealthy society exile? The healthy or the unhealthy?

Physician: The answer is a bit complicated.

Director: Why?

Physician: Because the sick society might banish the healthy, thinking the healthy are sick.

Director: Sick because they don't share the sick society's peculiar break with reality?

Physician: Yes.

Director: What madness.

Physician: At times the sane are an endangered species.

Director: What can we do when they are?

Physician: Try to win people over, one by one, to the cause.

27

Director: The cause?

Physician: A true view of the external world.

Director: But what about the internal world? Isn't there truth to be had in there?

Physician: Of course there is. But it can't be verified.

Director: Why not?

Physician: How would we go about it?

Director: We could ask questions and look for contradictions.

Physician: But what if I'm completely crazy yet never contradict myself?

Director: How is that possible?

Physician: Let's say I think I can fly, fly like a bird. And I never contradict myself on this score.

Director: Well, that's where the external comes in. One who never flew contradicts the claim that they can fly.

Physician: Are you sure?

Director: Of course. The reality contradicts the claim.

Physician: But what if the person claims to fly only by night, when none can see?

Director: Then why make the claim?

Physician: Yes. But, strictly speaking, it's not a contradiction, is it?

Director: It contradicts what we know about physics. And if you're going to do that, you need more than a simple assertion.

Physician: You have a point. But pointing out a contradiction, of whatever sort, is a delicate matter. People hate to be caught up.

Director: I don't.

Physician: Really? I don't know if I believe you.

Director: We can learn from our errors. And I want to learn.

Physician: Yes, but can't you see your errors on your own?

Director: Yes, but not always. And some of us never do.

Physician: True. And that's especially so when it comes to society.

Director: What do you mean?

Physician: Society almost never sees its own contradictions.

Director: But sometimes individuals see them?

Physician: Yes, and they have to be careful.

Director: Why?

Physician: Because society doesn't like being caught up!

Director: What happens when it is?

Physician: In the worst case? When society is sick? It persecutes those who show the error of its ways.

Director: So if society says A, B, and C are true, but you prove they're false....

Physician: You might be persecuted, yes.

Director: But how do you prove they're false?

Physician: How do you prove anything?

Director: I suppose you experiment.

Physician: Yes. And what do you do when your experiments support your hypothesis?

Director: You look for confirmation from your peers?

Physician: Right. But who are your peers?

Director: In a sick society? You tell me.

Physician: Your peers are the healthy, the relatively rare.

Director: So you ask the healthy to confirm what you conclude. And if they don't?

Physician: Then either you or they are wrong.

Director: But if they confirm?

Physician: Then you know.

28

Director: So we have to rely on others.

Physician: That's the only way. We can't exactly rely on society itself to prove to us it's wrong.

Director: Not even if we, to its face, catch it up in contradictions and lies?

Physician: That's a dangerous game.

Director: One the great minds play?

Physician: The great minds don't play.

Director: They don't ask uncomfortable questions?

Physician: Questions society will resent? They don't ask questions they know the answers to. They just state the facts.

Director: And a sick society won't resent hearing the facts? But how do we learn the facts?

Physician: We experiment, as we said.

Director: But how do we even know what to experiment on? Don't we have to do some asking around?

Physician: Well, true. We have to ask around.

Director: And when we ask around, and our questions aren't welcome, don't we begin to suspect something might be wrong?

Physician: Of course.

Director: And if, conversely, our questions are welcome, don't we begin to think there might be health?

Physician: Yes, a warm welcome is a good sign. But we have to be careful. Welcomes can deceive.

Director: True, and it's almost always good to be careful. But how can we best be careful?

Physician: By spending most of our time with a small band of healthy, proven friends.

Director: Friends who see the truth?

Physician: Friends who see the truth.

Director: But even among those who see, they don't always see every truth we see. Do they?

Physician: No, they don't.

Director: Not even if we try to prove our truth to them?

Physician: That doesn't always work.

Director: So there might be some discomfort even with our friends?

Physician: Yes. But they make up for it.

Director: How so?

Physician: They let us lean on them.

Director: And this is healthy.

Physician: Very healthy.

Director: Would you say the more healthy the society, the more people there are to lean on?

Physician: Yes, I would.

Director: And in the healthiest society, we can lean on everyone?

Physician: True, but that's an ideal never to be reached.

Director: Oh, I don't know. It might be possible.

Physician: What would that society be like?

Director: All would see and live up to truth.

Physician: But what if the truth is ugly?

Director: We still have to face it, no?

Physician: But what if the truth is ugly because of society?

Director: The society you can lean on? I don't understand.

Physician: What if society is, for instance, essentially belligerent? It makes enemies everywhere it goes, and wages constant external war to keep its internal peace?

Director: Hmm, yes. I see what you mean. But you're not saying internal peace is bad, are you?

Physician: What? No, of course not. I'm saying unending war is bad.

Director: War with whom?

Physician: What do you mean?

Director: What sort of enemies does this society fight? Healthy or unhealthy?

Physician: Why does that matter?

Director: Do you think it's good to fight the healthy?

Physician: No.

Director: How about the unhealthy?

Physician: Well, if I had to choose....

Director: What would be better than fighting the sick?

Physician: Trying to heal them.

Director: But can societies heal other societies?

Physician: That's a good question. I'm not sure they can.

29

Director: But let's say they can. Does the healing society aim to make the other perfectly well, or healthy enough?

Physician: Healthy enough.

Director: Healthy enough for what?

Physician: Avoiding war.

Director: Are we satisfied with that?

Physician: What more can we do? Make them healthy enough for happiness?

Director: Sure. But are we talking about the happiness of the society or the happiness of the individuals within the society?

Physician: The one implies the other.

Director: So what do we need to do?

Physician: We need to study the sick society first.

Director: And when we do, what do we see?

Physician: We'll probably see that it calls ill those who don't see things its way.

Director: And you can't be happy when you're deemed ill?

Physician: Of course not.

Director: Not even if you have a pleasant life?

Physician: How can you have a pleasant life if society is against you?

Director: Maybe you form a small society of your own.

Physician: You're talking about a band of friends?

Director: Yes. Happy?

Physician: I know what you're saying. But I find it hard to believe you can be happy with society's disapproval hanging over your head.

Director: Then we must heal this society. What do you think that would mean?

Physician: Making it so the society doesn't turn on its own.

Director: So the society will never deem anyone ill?

Physician: Well, certain people are certainly ill.

Director: Ill because they're actually sick and not because of their views?

Physician: Yes. We have to get this society to see things this way.

Director: See who's sick and well.

Physician: Right.

Director: And we'll know it's healed when we agree with what it sees?

Physician: That's the thing. We're assuming we know who's healthy or not. What if we don't?

Director: Then who are we to heal? But let's suppose we know. And let's suppose there are those in this society who are healthy but don't see things our way. That's possible, isn't it?

Physician: Of course it's possible.

Director: What do we do with them?

Physician: We try to persuade them.

Director: And if that fails?

Physician: We leave them alone.

Director: Why?

Physician: Why? Because a healthy society tolerates differing views!

Director: Even when it comes to sickness and health?

Physician: Even then.

30

Director: Coming from a doctor, that surprises me.

Physician: You don't think doctors know they can learn from different perspectives?

Director: Yes, but how widely varying are these perspectives?

Physician: As widely varying as can be.

Director: Really? Within two mostly like-minded societies?

Physician: Well, you have a point. The greatest differences in perspective usually come from outside a community like this.

Director: Outsiders see things with different eyes?

Physician: Yes, of course.

Director: So they can see sickness and health where their friends can't?

Physician: Sometimes, yes.

Director: How can an insider fail to see sickness?

Physician: Oh, it happens all the time.

Director: How?

Physician: Certain sicknesses come on gradually.

Director: And so you don't notice the change?

Physician: Exactly.

Director: Do you mind if I use a metaphor here?

Physician: Of course not.

Director: You're saying, basically, that if I sit in a room, and each night the lamp dims just a little, I might not notice a change until I'm in the dark?

Physician: Yes. But an outsider might see what's happening right away.

Director: They'll walk in, take one look, and ask why I'm working in a half lit room?

Physician: Precisely. They can help you realize what's happening to you.

Director: Then it's good to have outsiders around. But how might insiders fail to see health?

Physician: Health? They might have minor complaints. An ache here, a pain there — and this makes them forget that, overall, they're in wonderful health.

Director: So they let the minor complaints make them miss the big picture?

Physician: Yes, and that's where an outsider can help put things into perspective.

Director: You mean, they might say, 'Where I come from, people are suffering from terrible disease. You should be grateful.'

Physician: Sure, they'll say something like that — but with a bit more tact.

Director: And maybe they'll even invite some of the insiders to go to their society and see?

Physician: That would be a good lesson, yes.

Director: So our insiders have to be willing both to accept guests and to become guests.

Physician: Yes.

Director: Would you say this applies to every component of society, that they should all be willing to do this?

Physician: I certainly would.

Director: What's the most important component of society?

Physician: For most people? The family.

Director: So families should make a point of taking guests in and becoming guests to others?

Physician: If they hope to learn all they can, yes.

Director: What are other important components?

Physician: Schools.

Director: Is it the same with schools as with families?

Physician: Maybe even more so, because schools exist for learning.

Director: So we'll visit other schools and allow others to visit in turn?

Physician: Yes, and it's the same for all other components of society.

Director: Okay. But you've heard of closed societies?

Physician: Of course.

Director: They won't let us in.

Physician: That's true.

Director: Yes. And now that we're thinking of this, doesn't any society, no matter how open, have areas closed off from view?

Physician: Yes, and this is a problem.

Director: Why?

Physician: Those in a closed off area, a circle, are always at risk of becoming sick.

Director: Sick from what?

Physician: Stale air.

31

Director: What kind of illness results from this?

Physician: What kind? I'm not sure there's a name for it. But believe me — you know it when you see it.

Director: Does it go away if you leave the circle?

Physician: Usually, yes. But the one who leaves is in for a great big shock.

Director: From the fresh air?

Physician: No, the fresh air is a pleasant surprise. It's the light that shocks.

Director: How so?

Physician: It makes you see.

Director: See what?

Physician: The truth!

Director: You mean to say, the closed circle isolates itself from truth?

Physician: Of course!

Director: Is there a truth in particular?

Physician: Yes, the truth about who you are.

Director: Who do you think you are when you're in the circle?

Physician: Someone special.

Director: Physician, don't we all want to feel we're someone special?

Physician: Yes, but the circle tempts you to think you're more special than you are.

Director: Are you sure?

Physician: I am.

Director: But special in what respect?

Physician: Special in that you know.

Director: Know what?

Physician: Political things.

Director: Ah, I see. But do you actually know more about political things than those outside the circle?

Physician: You often do.

Director: And do you take what you know seriously?

Physician: Very seriously.

Director: But those who are outside the circle, but still manage to know — do they take what they know seriously?

Physician: When it's necessary to take it seriously, sure.

Director: So sometimes it's okay to play?

Physician: Of course! Lack of play makes you sick.

Director: And those in the circle don't often play?

Physician: I'd go so far as to say that when the circle is closed they never play.

Director: But surely they play.

Physician: What kind of play do they play?

Director: Serious play. A sort of high stakes poker, for instance.

Physician: Ha. That's the sort of 'play' those in closed circles love.

Director: So it's really not play in the sense you mean?

Physician: No, the sense I mean is simply having fun.

32

Director: What are you and I doing here today?

Physician: Talking while we hike.

Director: Are we taking the hike seriously?

Physician: Not too seriously, but seriously enough so we pay attention and don't get lost or hurt.

Director: And what about our talk? Serious?

Physician: Well, we've been talking about health.

Director: And health is a serious topic?

Physician: You have to ask?

Director: I'll take that as a yes. So our talk is in no way play?

Physician: I don't like to say that.

Director: Why not?

Physician: Because good conversation is a sort of game of the mind.

Director: And we're having fun with this game?

Physician: I am. Are you?

Director: I am. But there's something serious mixed with the fun.

Physician: Of course. It doesn't do to take the health of the body and mind too lightly.

Director: Nor the health of society.

Physician: True.

Director: Is that the limit of our game, body and mind and society, or is there another health we should be considering?

Physician: We should consider the health of the world.

Director: Do you mean this planet and the whole universe?

Physician: Let's hold off on taking on the health of the universe. But the planet? Yes, we should be concerned with its health.

Director: How do we know what makes for a healthy planet?

Physician: How do we know what makes for a healthy body?

Director: We use our minds.

Physician: Yes, we use our minds. And we use our minds to know what makes for a healthy planet. But how do we know what makes for a healthy mind? That's the question.

Director: We use our bodies.

Physician: Now you're really playing!

Director: Should we say the mind knows what makes for a healthy mind?

Physician: We should.

Director: And is that what's special about the mind? It regulates itself?

Physician: I think that's true.

Director: The mind regulates itself and everything else?

Physician: Yes.

Director: So a sick mind is a terrible crisis.

Physician: The worst sort of crisis.

Director: Would you say everyone in a healthy society has an interest when a mind grows sick?

Physician: I would.

Director: So what must everyone do?

Physician: I'm not sure what you have in mind.

Director: Mustn't they seek to regulate the sick mind just as they regulate their own?

Physician: Director, we don't regulate others' minds.

Director: What do we do?

Physician: We try to persuade them.

Director: So we say, 'Don't think like that. Think like this'?

Physician: Yes, something like that.

Director: And if that doesn't work?

Physician: I'll tell you what a sick society would do. It would say, 'Think this way or else.'

Director: But does that ever really happen?

Physician: Why wouldn't it?

Director: Because we can't read people's minds.

Physician: Not yet, at least.

Director: You have a point. But look at how things stand today. There is no reading of minds.

Physician: So what would a sick society do?

Director: Focus not on thoughts but deeds.

Physician: So it's, 'Think what you like, but do what I say'?

Director: Yes.

Physician: But what does this have to do with health?

Director: It's 'do what I say' because it's healthier that way.

Physician: That's what they'll say. But what if we're talking about a healthy society?

Director: I suppose it would encourage us to do healthy things.

Physician: And if we do these things, will our minds grow well?

Director: They should, don't you think?

Physician: I do. But what if they don't?

Director: Then we take the final step.

Physician: The final step for the mind? I can't wait to hear what this is. So what do we do?

Director: We wash the mind clean.

Physician: Brain washing? Ha, ha!

Director: Why do you laugh? What do you think 'brain washing' means?

Physician: To make people give up what they used to believe, and believe what you want.

Director: How can we tell what someone believes?

Physician: We can't.

Director: Oh, come on. Are you sure?

Physician: I suppose we can ask.

Director: And can we more than ask?

Physician: What would that mean?

Director: To have a full blown conversation with them.

Physician: Alright. I'll concede the point. But I think it would take many conversations. So how do you get them to stop thinking what they think?

Director: By convincing them it's false.

Physician: I don't think you know anything about brain washing, Director.

Director: Why? What am I doing wrong?

Physician: Before you can show them in a logical sort of way what they think is false, you have to get them to feel it's bad, feel it's wrong.

Director: You need moral force before you need reason?

Physician: To brain wash? Yes.

Director: And that's how you'd persuade? Through a sort of force?

Physician: Of course!

Director: And then you show them the new way of thought is good?

Physician: Good as good can be.

Director: I don't know, Physician. I don't think either of us knows anything about brain washing in this negative sense.

Physician: Negative sense? What's the positive sense?

Director: You know that positive sense as well as I. Regular washing is very important to health!

Physician: Ha, ha! Sure, if you rinse your mind with truth to wash away the mold. But negative brain washing washes away the truth.

Director: What truth?

Physician: What do you mean?

Director: What truth do the victims have? I mean, aren't they often terribly naive?

Physician: True.

Director: And if naive, not in touch with truth?

Physician: You have a point.

Director: So what gets washed away?

Physician: The beliefs they were taught.

Director: And what do they get in return?

Physician: New beliefs, and membership in a closed circle.

Director: But can't anyone join who washes and then believes the new beliefs?

Physician: Yes, I suppose.

Director: So is the circle really closed?

Physician: Tell me once you're in, and you try to get out.

33

Director: Well, I think that's enough about that. But I feel there's more we can say about mental health.

Physician: More we can say? Ha! Some people spend their whole lives saying things about mental health. And better them than those who think they've got it all figured out with nothing more to say!

Director: Yes. But surely we can figure some of it out. It's our highest imperative when it comes to health, no?

Physician: True.

Director: I wonder. Can you have a sort of closed circle in your mind?

Physician: I think that's an excellent question. And the answer is yes.

Director: What do we call the opposite of this?

Physician: Having an open mind.

Director: Is an open mind a healthy mind?

Physician: Of course it is.

Director: Then look at us! We've figured out all of mental health.

Physician: But what's an open mind? That's the trick.

Director: What trick? An open mind is willing to weigh and measure everything.

Physician: You mean, in order to know everything for what it is?

Director: Yes.

Physician: That's not what most people consider an open mind to be.

Director: What do they think?

Physician: They think an open mind is fair to all.

Director: If we weigh and measure accurately, aren't we fair?

Physician: I suppose. But let's be clear about what we're saying. All mental health boils down to knowing what things truly are. Yes?

Director: Yes.

Physician: You surprise me.

Director: Oh? Why?

Physician: You're usually not so categorical.

Director: Well, it seems you've caught me trying to take a shortcut.

Physician: How so?

Director: Knowing-what-things-truly-are is a very involved topic. We'd have to unpack it completely to see if what we're saying about mental health is true.

Physician: How long would that take?

Director: Longer than it takes to hike this trail and talk about health.

Physician: Then can we do that some other time?

Director: Of course. But where does that leave us?

Physician: It leaves me with a question. If we know full well what things are, but those things are terrible — are we mentally healthy then?

Director: More so than if we didn't know what those things are. But not everything is terrible.

Physician: Of course not.

Director: That said, even if things are mostly wonderful, there's still another difficulty here.

Physician: What is it?

Director: Suppose you know what ten things are, but most of society only knows what nine of those ten things are. What do you do?

Physician: You teach society about the tenth.

Director: Does it change if you know one hundred things and society still only knows nine?

Physician: No. You still try to teach.

Director: What if they don't want to learn?

Physician: You have to be persuasive.

Director: But what if they simply won't open their minds?

Physician: I guess you have seek out those who will.

Director: And if you're mistaken?

Physician: You mean, you try to teach the wrong people?

Director: Yes. Suppose they get angry.

Physician: Why would they get angry?

Director: Because they think they know more than they do.

Physician: And you contradict them in what they think they know?

Director: Yes.

Physician: But what do they think they know?

Director: They think they know, for instance, that wonderful things are terrible, and terrible things are wonderful.

Physician: And if you cross them concerning these things, they'll attack?

Director: I think they will. And what do you think they'll say? That you have an open mind?

Physician: Of course not. They'll say you're sick.

Director: But to be clear, they're not talking about clinically diagnosed sickness, are they?

Physician: No, they're talking about being 'sick' in the opposite sense in which they're 'well' because they 'know'.

Director: And they won't back down and say it's just a matter of opinion or taste?

Physician: They won't back down. And neither would I.

Director: Because you know to a certainty what certain things are.

Physician: Yes.

Director: And we're sure our enemies will say you're sick?

Physician: What else?

Director: They might say you're misguided, foolish, naive.

Physician: That would be the best they'd say.

Director: What would be the worst?

Physician: That I'm pernicious.

Director: That your views are harmful to society?

Physician: Yes.

Director: If they say this often enough, do you start to believe it's true?

Physician: That would be the danger for someone who's weak.

Director: But even for someone who's strong, if they hear it from when they're very young — might it not make them... ill?

Physician: That's a terrible thing you're saying.

Director: Terrible and true?

Physician: Terrible and true.

Director: So what can we do when we're young?

Physician: Not antagonize the 'knowers' to no good end.

Director: But if we see a good end?

Physician: We speak our mind. But even so, it's better to speak to open minds.

Director: So we have to learn the signs of openness?

Physician: We do.

Director: And learn the signs of minds that seem likely to open?

Physician: That, too.

Director: And don't tell them everything we know all at once?

Physician: No, just a little at a time. We don't want to scare them off.

Director: But if the mind we're dealing with closes up?

Physician: We have to let it close.

34

Director: Why?

Physician: Because a mind's opening isn't up to us.

Director: You mean, it can't be forced.

Physician: Correct.

Director: But a mind can be open about some things and closed about others, no?

Physician: Of course it can.

Director: So we'll find where it's open and take it from there?

Physician: Sounds like a plan.

Director: But what if we find a mind that's completely closed?

Physician: A completely closed mind would die. There's nothing we can do.

Director: Then let's work with what we can. How might we approach someone?

Physician: We might start with something fairly neutral. The health of the planet, say.

Director: In order to start there, we'd have to know something about the planet. Yes?

Physician: Certainly.

Director: How do we know something about the planet?

Physician: We know through science.

Director: Are people always open to science?

Physician: Always? Ha, ha. Hardly.

Director: When are they open?

Physician: When their beliefs aren't threatened.

Director: What about their interests?

Physician: That's an interesting question. Isn't the health of the planet, broadly speaking, in all of our interest?

Director: You would think. But there are those who take a narrow view.

Physician: Yes. And narrow views and the interests that go with them can wreck things for all.

Director: When we say 'narrow,' do we mean of closed mind?

Physician: We do.

Director: And tell me. Is it a fact that some of the narrow minded will never broaden their view?

Physician: It's a fact that most of the narrow minded will never broaden their view.

Director: So do we just give up?

Physician: No, we try. But only so much.

Director: And then what do we do?

Physician: We find other means.

Director: Means to do what?

Physician: Save the planet or whatever else we might be talking about!

Director: We're talking about making things healthy. But now I'm wondering. What if we're wrong? What if we're the narrow minded?

Physician: You mean we're speaking from our narrow interests and not the truth?

Director: Yes. What if?

Physician: I don't know, Director. Something that's truly in our interest is always aligned with truth.

Director: Can true interests clash?

Physician: I want to say no. But if they can, I think there's a great temptation.

Director: What temptation?

Physician: For one to call the other false.

Director: Meaning their interest isn't aligned with truth.

Physician: Yes. And they'll say that makes the false one sick.

Director: Is that what someone who's healthy does?

Physician: Of course not. Someone who does this is sick.

Director: What happens if the sick one is strong?

Physician: Strong? They might well smother the truth.

Director: The truth about the health of the other.

Physician: Yes, and their own bad health.

Director: What can the other one do?

Physician: Speak truth about the one who's sick.

Director: There's much we could say about this, isn't there?

Physician: I'm sure there is. But I don't like this line of conversation. Can't we talk about something else?

Director: Sure. What would you like to talk about?

Physician: You pick something.

Director: Okay. Let's talk about seriousness and play.

Physician: Ha! That sounds like a wonderful topic!

Director: Do you think seriousness and play are absolutes?

Physician: No. Haven't you ever heard someone say, 'I can't tell if you're being serious or not'?

Director: I have. And I've heard people say, 'I can't tell if you're playing or not.' Is it healthy to be ambiguous like that?

Physician: I think it can be.

Director: When?

Physician: When you're trying to figure out if someone's mind is open or not.

Director: If the mind is closed it will take what you say as play?

Physician: Yes.

Director: And if the mind is open it will take it seriously?

Physician: That's right.

Director: But isn't that wrong?

Physician: How so?

Director: The open mind should take it as both seriousness and play — because that's what it is.

Physician: True.

Director: But isn't there also something odd?

Physician: What do you have in mind?

Director: We're saying the closed minded are willing to play, or are at least open to play, or at least can recognize play.

Physician: But everyone can recognize play.

Director: Even the mentally ill?

Physician: Well, you have a point. Some of the mentally ill take seriousness as play, and play as seriousness.

Director: Hmm. Now I wonder. What happens if someone wants to play and you don't want to?

Physician: And they keep on trying to play? You get annoyed.

Director: And if someone wants to be serious and you don't want to?

Physician: You also get annoyed.

Director: Is the answer to be ambiguous?

Physician: But ambiguity gets annoying, too. In fact, it might even be more annoying.

Director: Why would it be more annoying?

Physician: Because it's maddening.

Director: Yes, but why is it maddening?

Physician: Because you don't know what to make of it!

Director: Make of it what it is — both seriousness and play.

Physician: But it makes you feel like you're being teased.

Director: Ah, teasing. Who can't stand to be teased?

Physician: In a friendly conversation? The overly serious.

Director: But the playful, they don't mind a good tease?

Physician: Of course not. They enjoy it.

Director: And do they enjoy a good bit of serious truth mixed in?

Physician: I'm sure some of them do.

Director: Those who aren't overly playful?

Physician: Yes, and I take your point. We need to be moderate when it comes to these things.

35

Director: Let me ask. When you take your endowed chair of health, and sit upon it in royal fashion, will you be playful or serious?

Physician: I'll be both.

Director: You'll be ambiguous?

Physician: Of course not. But I'll be serious at times, and playful at others.

Director: How will you know when to be which?

Physician: How does anyone know when to be which?

Director: Well, I like to think of myself as part of 'anyone', so I'll tell you what I do.

Physician: Please.

Director: I treat serious topics seriously, except when I'm trying to open a mind.

Physician: Yes, but I know you. You're always trying to open a mind!

Director: I'm trying to do that to you?

Physician: Of course! And I find it amusing.

Director: Why?

Physician: Because my mind is already open!

Director: But if I were to get serious with you?

Physician: That would be fine.

Director: Serious about a touchy subject?

Physician: What touchy subject do you have in mind?

Director: Trying to teach people health.

Physician: Teach people about health?

Director: No, teach people health.

Physician: I don't understand.

Director: Teaching health is like teaching kung fu.

Physician: Ha!

Director: You don't teach someone 'about' kung fu. You teach kung fu itself. Wouldn't you agree?

Physician: Yes, of course. And so it is with health?

Director: Yes, you teach them health.

Physician: So they'll be healthy.

Director: That's right.

Physician: Why is this a touchy subject?

Director: Because I doubt your employer will let you teach health.

Physician: You think they want me to teach students 'about health'?

Director: Yes.

Physician: Well, I'll just have to persuade them.

Director: Will you be playful or serious when you try to persuade?

Physician: I'll be serious, of course.

Director: Why not be ambiguous?

Physician: Because this is a serious conversation.

Director: What if they listen politely, then reveal their minds are closed on the matter?

Physician: Why would they care if I teach health?

Director: Tell me. Do you think the school is healthy?

Physician: Completely healthy? Faculty and students both? Of course not.

Director: If you try to teach a great big gang of students health, what happens if they storm around trying to teach health themselves throughout the school?

Physician: Throughout all the school? And not 'about health' but health itself? And they don't fully understand health? I think I see what you mean. Trouble.

Director: And there's more. Say you have a hundred students. How many do you think are fit to learn health?

Physician: Everyone is fit to learn health.

Director: But how many actually will?

Physician: Oh, I don't know. Fifty?

Director: Really?

Physician: Ten?

Director: Maybe. What happens when you fail the ninety and pass the ten?

Physician: More trouble.

Director: Right. So you see why I say this is a touchy topic?

Physician: Yes. But why can't I do both? Teach health and about health at once.

Director: That may be your only chance. But it'll be difficult, you know.

Physician: I do. But what choice do I have?

36

Director: So how do you see it? Will you teach 'health' as a subset of 'about health'?

Physician: I think it should be the other way round.

Director: Yes, but we're not dealing with 'should'. We're dealing with 'is'. The 'is' of your school and your chair.

Physician: But from my chair I want to change the 'is'.

Director: Then what will you do?

Physician: I will be forced, at least at first, to teach mostly 'about health'. But I will make it very clear that health itself is what it's all about.

Director: And then what?

Physician: I'll have generous office hours. And those who are interested in health itself will seek me out. And I will train them in kung fu.

Director: But will you tell them to be discreet when it comes to others on campus?

Physician: Yes, but they shouldn't be too discreet.

Director: What happens if they are?

Physician: Nothing changes!

Director: But do you want it to change like this? Suppose one of your mentees, one with a passionate interest in health, goes into math class and challenges the professor to a fight over how the class is being taught, about how healthy it is. Is that what you want?

Physician: Of course not.

Director: Don't even the best of the young sometimes do things like this?

Physician: Yes. But what can I do? This all sounds so hopeless.

Director: Because you won't know who to train?

Physician: No, because it will take forever and a day to make real change!

Director: Why?

Physician: Because I'll have to restrain my students!

Director: But what if 'real change' isn't what you want?

Physician: What? What in the world are you talking about? Why wouldn't I want a healthy campus, a healthy world?

Director: When people speak of 'real change', what do they usually mean?

Physician: Significant change.

Director: Isn't helping to improve the life of one of your students significant change?

Physician: Well, yes.

Director: But that's not enough for you? That's not real enough change?

Physician: Of course it's real. But I want more.

Director: How will you have more?

Physician: If I change ten lives, and they each change ten lives, and those others each change ten lives....

Director: Listen to you! You've got it all figured out. But who are those ten lives you'll change? Will any ten do?

Physician: No. They'll be special.

Director: What happens if you don't find and change those special ten?

Physician: What do you think might happen?

Director: You might grow desperate.

37

Physician: What would it take not to be desperate?

Director: What do the kung fu masters know?

Physician: I have no idea.

Director: They know that if the tradition carries on, if only in one, that's enough.

Physician: And if they don't find that one? Don't they get desperate about that?

Director: Why, no. You see, they're not afraid of death. And that applies to the death of the tradition, as well. But that's not to say they don't work as hard as they can to save it.

Physician: We have to work as hard as we can to save true health.

Director: Can you imagine anything worse than failing to save it?

Physician: No, I can't.

Director: I think there's something worse.

Physician: What?

Director: Corrupting it through despair.

Physician: Is that how it is with philosophy?

Director: Very much so. Philosophy has its own kung fu.

Physician: And its own tradition to carry on?

Director: In a way. But it would rather the tradition die pure, with a chance of rebirth, than have it live polluted by a cowardly craving for life. There. I've said something that sounds very serious.

Physician: Weren't you being serious?

Director: Who can say? But it sounds good, no? Something to share with your serious students?

Physician: And what should I share with my playful students?

Director: Why, everything! They can take it.

Physician: Because if things get too serious they'll make fun?

Director: A good safety valve to have. Good kung fu.

Physician: Yes, but will the playful fight the fight?

Director: Do you think the serious always will?

Physician: I do.

Director: Well, it's probably true.

Physician: But what about the playful?

Director: The playful might avoid the fight. That's why I favor the ambiguous.

Physician: Why not favor the serious?

Director: Because the serious sometimes mistake the fight.

Physician: In what sense?

Director: They fight the fight that doesn't need to be fought.

Physician: And the ambiguous know better?

Director: The ambiguous, those who can be serious and playful at once, always know when to fight.

Physician: Why?

Director: Because they have both perspective and resolve.

Physician: And this is healthy.

Director: This is very healthy. In fact, I'd say this is one of the healthiest things of all.

38

Physician: That's a tall claim.

Director: A tall claim for you.

Physician: How so?

Director: You need to teach perspective and resolve.

Physician: Resolve I can handle. But how do I teach perspective? Do I bring in foreign guests?

Director: Exposure to different perspectives is good. But it's not enough.

Physician: What does it take?

Director: Acting on what you learn from those perspectives. Making choices that affect you directly.

Physician: And discovering what each choice means?

Director: Yes.

Physician: But we're talking about my students' health, Director.

Director: How better to learn than when there's something at stake?

Physician: But the consequences of their choices might be serious!

Director: More reason for you to grade strictly. You don't want your students to think they know what they're doing when they don't. So fail the ninety and pass the ten.

Physician: You know I can't do that.

Director: Then do what you must. But what about the mentees who'll haunt your office hours? Will you let them face the consequences of their choices?

Physician: Let them? Once they choose, it's out of my control! The best I can do is influence the choice.

Director: How will you do that? Will you tell them what's best?

Physician: Well, then they never learn. I'll present them with options.

Director: All of them good?

Physician: Don't tell me you think I should include bad options, too.

Director: No, there's no need. They'll be able to come up with those all on their own.

Physician: That's why I need to earn their trust. So they tell me what they're thinking.

Director: And they might be thinking about something affecting their physical health?

Physician: Yes.

Director: Their mental health?

Physician: Of course.

Director: Societal health?

Physician: To a small extent? Certainly.

Director: The health of the planet?

Physician: Why not?

Director: Then this is remarkable.

Physician: In what sense?

Director: All of these things can be at risk when we learn health.

Physician: Yes, that's true.

Director: But then again, they're also at risk when we don't learn health.

Physician: Everything is always at risk?

Director: Isn't that life?

Physician: I suppose it is. So we may as well learn health!

Director: And when your students learn, what will they become?

Physician: A positive force in the world.

Director: So they'll attract the negative? Or don't you believe opposites attract?

Physician: You don't think the healthy attract the healthy?

Director: I don't think any of us are simply healthy. We're mixed, to some degree.

Physician: And so you think the bad parts of someone generally healthy will be attracted to the good parts of another? And the other way round?

Director: I don't know, Physician. The psychology of this gets deep very fast. But by and large? There might be some truth in here.

Physician: I agree. So tell me about a bad part of you that attracts me to you as a friend.

Director: A bad part? Here's one. I don't believe in what your school tries to teach. Or is that a good part of me?

Physician: Ha, ha!

Director: What's a bad part of you?

Physician: I don't believe in what my school tries to teach, either! But what is it we don't believe?

Director: We don't believe in teaching about the thing. Instead we'd teach the thing itself.

Physician: You know, I'm going to run into plenty of professors who won't understand that distinction.

Director: They think they're teaching the thing itself when they really only teach about?

Physician: Yes. They're blind when it comes to this.

Director: It's funny you should say that. Do you think it's unhealthy to be blind?

Physician: Yes, but it's complicated.

Director: How so? Healthy eyes see, no?

Physician: Of course. But the blind are blind through no fault of their own. So it becomes a moral question at this point.

Director: Moral? Health is a question of morality?

Physician: Of course it is!

Director: How so?

Physician: Suppose you grow up in what we call a highly developed society, with a more or less healthy diet. You'll be in fairly good health, yes?

Director: Odds are, at least.

Physician: Fair enough. But what about someone who starves in a little developed society? They'll be in fairly bad health, no?

Director: Probably so, yes.

Physician: So do you see?

Director: See what?

Physician: See that it's a moral question!

Director: Because something might be done about starvation?

Physician: Yes!

Director: But nothing, yet, can be done about being blind.

Physician: It's still a moral issue, because if only we try we might be able to figure out a way to help.

Director: Morality is about help?

Physician: Yes, definitely so.

Director: And that's one reason why you want to help your students learn health?

Physician: Very much so.

Director: And this moral impulse of yours is a positive?

Physician: What could be more positive?

Director: I don't know. But let's hope a great big negative doesn't come along and hurl itself at you.

39

Physician: Oh, forget about positive and negative. Let's focus on healing.

Director: Can healing ever be a negative?

Physician: I see you haven't forgotten.

Director: It's hard to forget. But can it?

Physician: No, healing is always a positive.

Director: Because healing leads to health.

Physician: Of course.

Director: And health is always a positive.

Physician: Can there be any doubt?

Director: What if a tyrant is healthy? Is that a positive?

Physician: I don't believe a tyrant can have mental health.

Director: To the extent a tyrant has mental health he or she can't be a tyrant?

Physician: I think that puts it well.

Director: So a tyrant is always sick.

Physician: Yes, absolutely.

Director: If we heal a tyrant, does the tyranny go away?

Physician: It does.

Director: Hmm. How easy is it to heal a tyrant?

Physician: Not very easy at all.

Director: Because a tyrant is completely negative?

Physician: Well, he or she certainly isn't positive. But, come on! Can't we just forget about positive and negative?

Director: Sorry. Instead of 'negative' let's say 'bad'. Is a tyrant, a tyrant proper, all bad?

Physician: Isn't he or she so by definition?

Director: And the wholly bad are very hard to heal?

Physician: Mentally speaking? Yes, of course.

Director: What's the first step to healing a tyrant? And you know, we're not just talking about heads of state. We're talking about petty tyrants, too.

Physician: Yes, and it makes sense to talk about them all — because fundamentally they're the same.

Director: What's the first step?

Physician: You need to show them you, too, have force.

Director: Because that's all a tyrant respects?

Physician: Yes.

Director: But what if we don't have much force?

Physician: We all have force. Moral force.

Director: And tyrants respect moral force? You haven't met many tyrants, have you?

Physician: Oh, I've met my share.

Director: And moral force was enough with them?

Physician: Well, it was moral force with the threat of something else.

Director: Physical force?

Physician: No. Political force.

Director: Political force? What's that?

Physician: What a healthy society can bring to bear.

Director: And tyrants come to power when society lacks this force?

Physician: Yes. Society must always exercise force to keep would-be tyrants at bay.

Director: And the only way a society stays healthy enough to maintain this force, is if everyone strives for their own health?

Physician: That's exactly the way.

Director: So when we fight for our own health, we're fighting for something more.

Physician: Yes.

Director: Because if everyone has health, society can't be sick.

Physician: We're talking about mental health, right?

Director: Right.

Physician: Then no, society can't be sick.

40

Director: Is there a way to ensure it stays healthy?

Physician: The only way is for everyone to be on the lookout for sickness, sickness in the most general sense, even in its earliest stage.

Director: And seek to treat it right away?

Physician: Yes, regardless if it poses no immediate threat.

Director: What if the sick don't want to be treated?

Physician: A healthy society would tell them there's no choice.

Director: A healthy society leaves you with no choice?

Physician: If it wants to stay healthy? Yes.

Director: But what about the rare case?

Physician: What rare case?

Director: The case of the wise.

Physician: Why would they need to be treated?

Director: Don't you know? There's much that can go wrong with the wise.

Physician: You mean, the wise are often sick?

Director: Yes, as often as any others are sick.

Physician: So what can we do?

Director: Craft a treatment appropriate to them.

Physician: I know what that treatment might be.

Director: What?

Physician: For them to teach!

Director: Teaching will make them well?

Physician: When you're wise, when you truly have something to share, teaching heals.

Director: We're saying a healthy society forces the wise to teach?

Physician: Of course!

Director: Does it force the less-than-wise to learn?

Physician: Oh, you can't force that. It doesn't work. You have to open up to learning on your own.

Director: And you don't have to open up to teaching on your own?

Physician: Well....

Director: Well indeed. But suppose we do force our wise ones to teach. What will they teach?

Physician: You're wondering whether they'll teach 'the thing itself'?

Director: Yes.

Physician: Well, let's be serious. There's no forcing that.

Director: Why not?

Physician: Because it defeats the purpose.

Director: The purpose?

Physician: It takes freedom to teach the thing.

Director: Why?

Physician: You're just giving me a hard time.

Director: No, I really want to know what you think. Why freedom?

Physician: Let's forget about wisdom and go back to health. There is no health without freedom.

Director: Mental health, you mean?

Physician: Yes. Do you think it's true?

Director: Some say a free mind is the very definition of health.

Physician: Yes. And you can never be forced to teach others how to be free, nor can you force a mind to learn to be free.

Director: Then what can we do?

Physician: We can persuade the healthy to show the sick what freedom can be. Or we can remind the sick of how they once felt — if they had ever been free.

41

Director: 'If they had ever been free.' You know, some believe we're all born free, but many of us lose our freedom throughout our lives, even at a very young age.

Physician: Yes, but I believe we're all born unfree and have to learn how to be free, have to learn how to fight to be free.

Director: And freedom is always healthy?

Physician: Of course.

Director: What else is always healthy?

Physician: Well, nothing. Or nothing I can think of right now.

Director: Will a free mind make the body healthy?

Physician: I think it can, over time.

Director: And will a healthy body make the mind free?

Physician: It can contribute to it, support it. But there are many with healthy bodies and unfree minds.

Director: So the mind is still the thing.

Physician: Yes.

Director: Even if we manage to make our bodies perfect through technology, it doesn't matter much unless our minds are free?

Physician: Absolutely.

Director: Can we use technology to make our minds free?

Physician: Suppose we could. What's the quality of that freedom?

Director: What do you mean?

Physician: I mean we haven't earned it.

Director: You'd turn down a freedom that's free?

Physician: Ha! You know I would. And so would you.

Director: Freedom must always be won.

Physician: Yes, and each generation has to win it all over again — or it's lost.

Director: Hmm. You know what I wonder? What would be your use as a teacher if all your students came to you already free, their battles already won?

Physician: Yes, but no one is perfectly free.

Director: You mean we all have something to learn?

Physician: Don't you agree?

Director: What can we learn?

Physician: How to be even more free.

Director: And what makes us even more free?

Physician: For example? Having fewer prejudices.

Director: And that means learning not to believe something we believe?

Physician: Right.

Director: What about the opposite?

Physician: Learning to believe something we don't believe?

Director: Yes. Can that make us even more free?

Physician: No doubt it can.

Director: What's an example?

Physician: Learning to believe in yourself.

Director: You'll teach your inner circle of students that belief?

Physician: I'll teach all of my students that belief!

Director: But what if 'yourself' is stuffed full of prejudice? Should you believe in it then?

Physician: You need to think your prejudices through in order to arrive at the true you.

Director: And when you believe in that 'you', you're free?

Physician: Yes.

Director: So we think in order to arrive at the belief that makes us well.

Physician: Exactly.

Director: But does thinking always lead to health?

Physician: Do you have any doubt?

Director: I do. That's why I asked.

Physician: I don't believe you.

Director: You don't believe I doubt? Why not?

Physician: How could you, of all people, possibly doubt that thinking makes for health?

Director: Think of it this way. Have you ever tried to do something very hard, something exhausting?

Physician: Of course I have.

Director: Can you see how if you grew exhausted enough, you might become sick?

Physician: I can. And we talked about this, about overdoing it.

Director: Well, thinking is sometimes very hard, exhausting.

Physician: And so thinking sometimes makes us sick? Okay. I can see how that's possible. But that doesn't mean thinking is bad.

Director: No, I'm not saying thinking is bad. But what I'm wondering is whether thinking is more important than health.

42

Physician: Doesn't thinking always lead, beyond whatever initial sickness, to greater health?

Director: I don't know.

Physician: But if thinking doesn't ultimately lead to health, why in the world would you want to think?

Director: Because you just can't resist.

Physician: Oh, that's ridiculous.

Director: Is it?

Physician: Yes!

Director: Let's look at health for a moment. Can you imagine anyone saying, 'I just can't resist being healthy'?

Physician: Well, there are many enthusiasts. But no, that doesn't sound like something someone would say.

Director: Don't people often say, 'I have to will myself to be healthy'? 'I force myself to go to the gym'? 'I struggle to resist my appetite'? And so on?

Physician: You have a point. But what does that have to do with thought being irresistible?

Director: Don't you sometimes hear people say, 'I can't help but think...'?

Physician: Yes, but that's just a turn of phrase.

Director: But it means even if they don't want to think something, they do. Don't you think that happens?

Physician: Alright, yes. It happens.

Director: And it means the thought was irresistible. No?

Physician: I'll concede the point.

Director: Now here's the thing. Is it only certain people who can't resist, or is it that no one can resist?

Physician: Oh, I think many people can resist thought.

Director: But they pay a price?

Physician: You want me to say resistance sickens them?

Director: Does it?

Physician: For the sake of argument, I'll agree.

Director: How do they resist their thoughts?

Physician: They will the thoughts away.

Director: So without a will, thought comes freely? We simply can't resist and therefore open up and love to think?

Physician: You know that's not how it works. We don't always love what we can't resist.

Director: Don't we? I can't resist chocolate because I love chocolate. I can't resist thought because I love thought.

Physician: I don't know, Director.

Director: What do you love?

Physician: I love helping people.

Director: Let's examine this a bit. With chocolate, if you eat too much, you'll get sick. Yes?

Physician: Yes, and if you think too much, you, too, will get sick.

Director: Ah, but what's too much? But if you help people too much?

Physician: There's no such thing.

Director: If you were a parent, trying to help your child learn to ride a bike, and you never let go, isn't that helping too much?

Physician: I suppose.

Director: Of course it is! You know that.

Physician: So you're saying when I teach, I need to learn when to let go.

Director: Yes.

Physician: But letting go is helping.

Director: I won't object to your looking at it that way.

Physician: You don't think that's the right way to look at it?

Director: When you let go, you help no more.

Physician: Okay, that is, strictly speaking, true. But tell me this. What if they, my students, come back after I let go, so to speak, and ask for more help?

Director: Ah, that's very difficult. The answer depends on how much you admire them.

Physician: How so?

Director: If you admire them a great deal, you refuse to help.

Physician: Because you know they're strong enough to do it on their own?

Director: Yes. And for the others? You simply might have misjudged and need to hold on a bit more.

Physician: But I don't like where this leads.

Director: What do you mean?

Physician: Let's say I have a student I greatly admire, so much so that I'm certain they don't need my help at all. What then?

Director: Don't you think it would be a pleasure to have a student like that?

Physician: Yes, but I'll never get to help!

Director: Maybe helping isn't what you love.

Physician: What do you think I love?

Director: Admiring the health of others.

Physician: You really think that's what I love? But it's so... passive!

Director: Well, maybe you love both — helping and admiring.

Physician: And do you admire the thoughts of others?

Director: I certainly do. So it's true with me, too. I love both — thinking and admiring thought.

43

Physician: Yes, but I wonder if we can reduce it all down to something very basic.

Director: I should tell you, my friend — I'm wary of grand reductions.

Physician: But what if the reduction is true?

Director: What do you have in mind?

Physician: Health, mental health, can be reduced to your mind doing what it loves.

Director: Have you forgotten already? We said what I love, thinking, can make you sick.

Physician: Yes, but I mean to say that mental health is the mind doing what it loves without doing it too much, without getting sick.

Director: Moderation, in other words.

Physician: Yes, exactly.

Director: Hmm. Tell me. If you're dying from thirst in a desert, should you be moderate in crawling toward the oasis?

Physician: No, but is that really a good example?

Director: Well, let's look at it this way. Have you ever wanted to know something, know it so badly you didn't care about the cost, you just had to know?

Physician: Well, of course I've wanted to know. But did I disregard the cost to my health? I have to be honest. No.

Director: Then it might be hard for you to understand how thinking is, at times, for me.

Physician: These are the times you get sick?

Director: Sometimes. But sometimes I'm lucky and my strength holds out. The point is that I'm willing to take the risk.

Physician: You're forcing me to wonder about my own love of healing.

Director: I thought you love to help.

Physician: How does someone like me help best but by healing?

Director: So is it heal or die? Have you ever had to crawl through a desert on your way toward the oasis of health?

Physician: I have.

Director: Would you do it again?

Physician: Without any doubt.

Director: Because healing is simply your way of life?

Physician: Simply and precisely so.

Director: But has your love ever made you sick?

Physician: I'm sick when I fail.

Director: Because you tried with all your might?

Physician: Yes.

Director: Are you ever sick when you try so hard and succeed?

Physician: Sometimes I am, but it's easier to take.

Director: Then it seems we have much in common.

Physician: I'm going to have to teach this, you know.

Director: What will you teach?

Physician: That the healing of others can be more important than your health.

Director: It's interesting you should say that.

Physician: Oh? Why?

Director: I'll explain it this way. When I'm in my desert, I think. And the oasis I arrive at is knowledge. So we can say I'm thinking for the sake of knowledge, no? Similarly, we can say you're healing for the sake of health, the health of others or even your own.

Physician: Yes, but what are you trying to say?

Director: If it's healing for the sake of health, is health the more important thing?

Physician: The health of the other, yes. Just as when it's thinking for the sake of knowledge, knowledge is more important than thought.

Director: But I'm not so sure that's so.

Physician: Why, are they equally important?

Director: Some might say that's how it is. But we might also say it's health for the sake of healing, and knowledge for the sake of thought.

Physician: That doesn't sound right.

Director: Haven't you ever heard that the process is more important than the product?

Physician: I've heard that the journey is more important than the destination. Is that what you mean? But in my case, the case of healing and health, I'm not so sure I like that idea.

Director: Which will you give precedence when you teach? Healing or health?

Physician: Well, I am the chair of health. But what about you?

Director: Me? I'm glad for knowledge, very glad — make no mistake. But thinking is what I love. And I'm not always in the desert.

44

Physician: Let's consider thinking and health a little bit more.

Director: Alright. If you have no health, none at all, can you think?

Physician: No.

Director: And if you never think, not at all, can you be healthy?

Physician: Ha, ha. I sometimes think you can!

Director: But seriously, is that what you think?

Physician: No, no thought no health.

Director: So they depend on each other, at least to some degree. Is that fair to say?

Physician: Yes, it's fair.

Director: Then I wonder what happens if we say this.

Physician: Say what?

Director: That if we want a great deal of thinking, we need a great deal of health.

Physician: I believe it.

Director: And if we want a great deal of health...

Physician: ...we need a great deal of thinking.

Director: What do you think?

Physician: It doesn't hold up.

Director: Why not?

Physician: Because I've had plenty of healthy patients I would hardly call thinkers.

Director: But how would you know?

Physician: Oh, Director, it's obvious.

Director: How do we know when someone thinks?

Physician: They're able to give an account of what they think.

Director: No, I don't agree. That's a skill in its own right.

Physician: But then how do we know they're thinking?

Director: We know by what they don't say.

Physician: Yes, but then the ideal is being mute!

Director: Of course we're not talking about mutes. But if someone holds a normal conversation, but is silent concerning certain things that come up, doesn't that make you think?

Physician: This is your love of thought. Anything would make you think, even silence!

Director: Yes, but I might have good reason to think. And if good reason to think, good reason to ask.

Physician: Ask what?

Director: Ask the silent one what they think.

Physician: About the 'certain things' that came up?

Director: Yes. And not in an aggressive way. But in a gentle way, away from everyone else.

Physician: And you believe that based on what they say, you'll know how much they think?

Director: Yes.

Physician: Well, you might have a point.

Director: So we shouldn't judge how much another thinks until we've had the chance to see?

Physician: I have to agree. But are you sure you're not looking for an account?

Director: I'm just looking for a friendly little chat.

Physician: So if doctors chat with their patients, they will be able to see how well thinking correlates with health?

Director: Yes, but they have to be sure to chat about those 'certain things' that come up.

Physician: But how will they come up?

Director: The doctors will have to bring them up.

Physician: Ha, ha! You're just trying to get me into trouble, aren't you?

Director: Why, no. I'm counting on you to get yourself into trouble. And that, my friend, might be the only way — you'll learn to love to think.

45

Physician: Ha, ha. Ever joking. But tell me this. Can't you be born into trouble?

Director: Isn't it your opinion we're all born into trouble to the extent we're born unfree?

Physician: It is. And it's unfortunate. Because if you get yourself into trouble, you'll have some idea of how to get back out. But if you're born into trouble, it's much harder to find your way.

Director: Always? Maybe so. But let's look at a few examples. What's one way of getting yourself into trouble?

Physician: Aside from bringing up 'certain things'? There are a million ways.

Director: How about taking on overwhelming debt?

Physician: That's certainly trouble.

Director: What's the way out?

Physician: You either find a way to pay it off over time or declare yourself bankrupt.

Director: Is it easy to know these are the ways?

Physician: Of course.

Director: And what's a way, aside from being unfree, of being born into trouble?

Physician: I suppose your family could be in the mob.

Director: Organized crime? Yes, that's trouble. So what's the way out?

Physician: To have nothing to do with what they do.

Director: Then isn't that also easy to know?

Physician: I don't think it is.

Director: Why not?

Physician: Because the way of your family is all you know.

Director: Just as when you're born unfree that's all you know?

Physician: True.

Director: So, in either case, you have to learn there's another way.

Physician: Yes, and learning that way is hard.

Director: Now tell me. What effect on our health does being in trouble have?

Physician: Well, it can't be good.

Director: Why not?

Physician: Because your trouble weighs on you.

Director: What does that mean?

Physician: It causes stress. And stress is very bad for the body.

Director: But also bad for the mind, assuming again we treat body and mind as distinct?

Physician: It's probably worse for the mind than body.

Director: Then we should do everything we can not to be in trouble.

Physician: I love how you make the obvious sound profound.

Director: Then you'll really love this. You, Physician, must help get and keep your students out of trouble. For the sake of their health.

Physician: I hadn't thought about that. But I think you're right!

Director: I speak to your love of helping others — and look at you! You're excited.

Physician: Of course I am! More opportunity to help. I love it.

Director: So how will you help?

Physician: I'll help them see the way out.

Director: And when they see?

Physician: They have to act. And that's what's really hard.

Director: Can you help them here?

Physician: I can encourage them and keep them honest.

Director: And by 'honest' you mean something like holding them to task?

Physician: Yes.

Director: Is it healthy to be honest like this?

Physician: Of course it is.

Director: And if we're honest, we'll stay out of trouble?

Physician: It's much more likely we will.

Director: So we're likely to suffer less from stress.

Physician: That's right.

Director: Do we also have a better chance at being strong?

Physician: Absolutely.

Director: Why?

Physician: Because fighting stress only saps our strength. But in staying on task, we grow strong.

Director: What's the point of growing strong?

Physician: You're not seriously asking me that, are you?

Director: I'm asking if it's strength for its own sake.

Physician: It's strength for the sake of health, as we've said.

Director: Yes, we said strength belongs to health. But what if health belonged to strength?

Physician: Strength would be the end? No, that doesn't make sense.

Director: Why not?

Physician: Because strength, without an object to apply itself to, is nothing. And when you do have an object, that's your end. Do you see what I mean?

Director: I do. But haven't you heard people say the free exercise of strength, no matter the object, is the true end?

Physician: I've heard them. And I always think how empty an existence that would be. But now you make me wonder. Didn't you say the end of health is to enjoy it?

Director: Let me guess. You think enjoying health is an empty existence, too. You think there should be something beyond mere enjoyment as our end.

Physician: Now that I think of it? Yes. And I worry for you.

Director: Worry? Why?

Physician: Because I think you see thought as your end. And no matter how you love it, that's as empty as it gets.

46

Director: Aren't you being a little too harsh? But don't worry, Physician. That's not my end.

Physician: Then what is?

Director: I was hoping that might become clear in talking with you.

Physician: Ha! You mean you don't know? But we need to know, always know! Surely you believe we can know the purpose of things.

Director: I'm sure we can posit a purpose.

Physician: So what happens if we posit health?

Director: As the purpose of life? Aside from enjoying it? We may well have more healthy people.

Physician: But that's not what you want?

Director: Who doesn't want more healthy people?

Physician: But what do you really want? More thinkers? More philosophers?

Director: Philosophy as the purpose of life? But what if philosophy questions why we have to have a purpose at all?

Physician: If it does, philosophy will find our health suffers when we lack purpose.

Director: So it's purpose for the sake of health.

Physician: Yes.

Director: But then why not take the next step and say health is the purpose?

Physician: So it's health for the sake of health?

Director: Do you see anything wrong with that?

Physician: You're the one who should tell me!

Director: Well, I do see a problem here.

Physician: What problem?

Director: If that's the way it is, we'd never do anything that might jeopardize our health.

Physician: Name such a thing.

Director: Imagine you have a sick child. You stay up nights to nurse her or him back to health. You know you're not getting enough sleep to stay healthy, and we'll say the child's illness is contagious.

Physician: But that only proves that health is the most important thing! The health of the child.

Director: And would you extend that?

Physician: How so?

Director: Say you're a scientist working yourself to death in order to save the planet.

Physician: Sure, why not? Once again, health is what's important. Just not necessarily my own health.

Director: You'd never hear me say that about philosophy.

Physician: What do you mean?

Director: I'd never say, 'Thinking is what's important — but not necessarily my thinking.'

Physician: Because if thinking is important, it's important for you.

Director: Yes. But we're not saying the same for health.

Physician: That's because of love. Love for the sick child. Love for the planet and those who live here.

Director: Is love the purpose of life?

Physician: I think it is! What's more important than love?

Director: Nothing. But I think it gets complicated here.

Physician: In what way?

Director: Let me give you an example. Have you ever fallen in love with someone you shouldn't have fallen in love with?

Physician: Well....

Director: Have you?

Physician: I have. My best friend's girlfriend, a long time ago. But what's your point?

Director: If love is the most important thing, we should always follow love.

Physician: Okay, but what we're talking about in this example is infatuation, not love.

Director: How can you tell the two apart?

Physician: Love endures.

Director: And infatuation is fleeting? Always?

Physician: It doesn't endure like love.

Director: But can you know it's fleeting at the time?

Physician: Not at the time, no.

Director: Then how do you know not to follow it?

Physician: You just know. And I know you know.

Director: How do you know that?

Physician: Because I would bet you, too, have fallen in love like this — or been infatuated, I should say. Have you?

Director: I've known infatuation.

Physician: So when you feel it, what do you do about it?

Director: Would you believe me if I told you I do nothing but wait and see?

Physician: No. But would you be waiting to see if it's love?

Director: Yes. And do you know what else I look for?

Physician: I have no idea.

Director: Health. If it turns out to be love, don't you think it must be healthy love?

Physician: Of course I do. But how do you know if love is healthy?

Director: It often helps to have some experience with unhealthy love, so you know the difference.

Physician: What's the most unhealthy love you've ever had?

Director: One that seemed healthy but wasn't.

Physician: And so you didn't know what to do?

Director: Yes, I didn't know whether to stay or go.

Physician: But eventually you knew. You knew you had to break free.

Director: At the simplest level, that's true. Still, this points to a problem.

Physician: What problem?

Director: Breaking free can be good. But what happens if we only ever break free?

Physician: You mean, what happens if we never find a healthy love?

Director: That's what I mean. In that case, do we have no purpose in life?

Physician: Well, there are other kinds of healthy love.

Director: What are they?

Physician: Love for family. Love for friends. Love for the world.

Director: And you can find purpose with any of them?

Physician: Yes, of course.

Director: And you can be healthy with any of them?

Physician: Without a doubt.

Director: Hmm.

Physician: What is it?

Director: I'm not sure your list is exhaustive. And I wonder about health.

Physician: How so?

Director: Can love make you healthy if you're not?

Physician: Physically healthy? Sometimes, yes — amazingly so.

Director: And what about mentally?

Physician: Miracles happen here, too — and even more often.

Director: But should we depend on miracles?

Physician: Of course not. We need to make ourselves as healthy as can be — so we bring our best to love.

47

Director: Well, we're past the halfway point of the trail. How are you holding up?

Physician: I feel great!

Director: Good! So tell me. How do we make ourselves as healthy as can be? Physically, everyone has advice. Eat this, exercise that. But what about mentally?

Physician: It's much the same, if in a different way.

Director: Eat this, exercise that? So what's the eating?

Physician: Experience.

Director: And the exercising?

Physician: Thinking.

Director: And just to be clear, we experience something when we read a book, for instance. Yes?

Physician: Yes, we do.

Director: What happens if we experience but don't think?

Physician: We grow unhealthy.

Director: Is it better not to experience at all?

Physician: Then we starve.

Director: So what do you recommend, doctor?

Physician: A moderate amount of experience coupled with a moderate amount of thought.

Director: But what about a great amount of experience with a great amount of thought? Wouldn't that be best?

Physician: Maybe for some.

Director: What about little experience with a great amount of thought?

Physician: Well, I suppose you'd be sure to digest your experience thoroughly.

Director: Thinking as digesting. I like that. But....

Physician: But we should stress that it's best to take in high quality food.

Director: High quality experience? How do we acquire that?

Physician: We have to have good taste.

Director: Is good taste something we learn or is it something we simply have?

Physician: It's something we simply have, but have to learn we have it.

Director: That sounds profound.

Physician: Since you mentioned it — do you think it's healthy to be profound?

Director: As opposed to being superficial?

Physician: Yes. Which is better?

Director: I suppose it all depends.

Physician: On what?

Director: On what you're dealing with.

Physician: So if I'm dealing with superficial things, it's best if I'm superficial?

Director: Doesn't that seem best?

Physician: It does. Because if you try to be profound, you'll be disappointed, frustrated.

Director: Enough so that you become ill?

Physician: If you keep it up for a long enough time? Sure.

Director: And does it follow that it's healthy to be profound when dealing with the profound?

Physician: It does, as only seems fitting.

Director: Then health is about the appropriate, the fitting?

Physician: Yes, I think it is.

Director: Suppose we have a friend who's being inappropriate.

Physician: You mean, for instance, they're being superficial with things profound?

Director: Yes. What should we do?

Physician: Maybe if we're profound our example will help.

Director: Maybe. But do you think our friend will also need a lesson on how to be superficial with things inherently superficial?

Physician: Ha, ha. Probably not. But what's an example of something inherently superficial?

Director: Judging a book by its cover. What do you think?

Physician: I think that's a very good example. Forming profound judgments based on a cover is foolish. But what's something that's inherently profound?

Director: That's a harder question.

Physician: Why?

Director: I'm not sure what makes something profound.

Physician: Maybe it's having much to digest?

Director: But are you really happy with that notion?

Physician: Why wouldn't I be?

Director: Look at it this way. If you eat something simple, an apple, that's not much to digest, right?

Physician: Right.

Director: But what if you eat a bushel of apples?

Physician: That's a lot to eat.

Director: And therefore profound?

Physician: No, I wouldn't say that.

Director: Why not?

Physician: Because profundity, like experience, is about quality, not quantity.

Director: So what's the quality?

Physician: Being hard to think through.

Director: Ah. Let's consider an example. Poetry. Can it be profound?

Physician: Of course it can, and it regularly is.

Director: What makes it hard to think through?

Physician: Some poetry is notorious for not telling you everything. You get unexplained sentiments and fragments of thoughts.

Director: So, in a poem like this, how do we think these things through?

Physician: If the sentiments and fragments support one another, we might be able to put two and two together and arrive at four.

Director: And if they don't support one another?

Physician: We might conclude that the poem is nonsense.

Director: Is that a thinking through?

Physician: If it's truly nonsense? Yes, I think that's a thinking through. We see it for what it is.

Director: But isn't there often a temptation to say the profound is nonsense, before we've thought it through?

Physician: I agree. It's easy to dismiss.

Director: And looking at it the other way, doesn't a lot of nonsense pass for the profound?

Physician: Regularly.

Director: Why do you think that is?

Physician: Because people don't make the effort to add things up. When something seems hard to figure, they just throw up their hands and say it's profound.

Director: They're not willing to think it all the way through.

Physician: Right.

Director: But if they do think it through?

Physician: Well, if they find it makes good sense —

Director: Hold on. What does 'makes good sense' mean?

Physician: It means the thing in question clearly points to a difficult truth. And this is profound.

48

Director: What's the opposite of a difficult truth?

Physician: A simple truth.

Director: What happens if we fail to grasp simple truths?

Physician: We become ill. Do you agree?

Director: I couldn't agree more.

Physician: But what happens if we fail to grasp a difficult truth?

Director: It depends.

Physician: On what?

Director: On whether it's a truth for you.

Physician: If it's for you and you fail to grasp it, you become ill?

Director: Yes.

Physician: Can you give an example?

Director: How about war?

Physician: But everyone should grasp the truth about war.

Director: Why?

Physician: Because then we'd have fewer wars!

Director: And how do we learn the difficult truth about war?

Physician: By living through one.

Director: So we want everyone to live through a war so they can grasp its truth?

Physician: Well, I'm not sure I'd wish that on everyone.

Director: Yes, and now I'm having doubts about what I said.

Physician: What doubts?

Director: Maybe the truth about war isn't difficult at all. Terrible as it is, it might be very simple.

Physician: And simple truths belong to all?

Director: I want to say yes. But then something occurs to me. Is it possible that what's simple for you is difficult for me?

Physician: I suppose it is.

Director: And what's simple for me might be difficult for you?

Physician: Yes.

Director: Do we both have to grasp both those truths?

Physician: Well, that's the question. How do we know which truths are ours to grasp?

Director: We walk away.

Physician: What? What do you mean?

Director: We give it some space and see how we feel.

Physician: And if we start to feel sick?

Director: We know we need to go back.

Physician: Okay. But there are times when we can't walk away.

Director: Then it seems we have no choice but to grasp.

Physician: What does it mean to grasp?

Director: To understand.

Physician: And what does it mean to understand?

Director: To know.

Physician: And what does it mean to know?

Director: To have mastered.

Physician: How do we master a truth?

Director: We look it right in the eye and stare it down.

Physician: We tame the truth?

Director: Ha, ha. Maybe so.

Physician: So what happens when the truth is tame?

Director: We can live with it like a pet.

Physician: Oh, now you're just being ridiculous.

Director: Don't you like pets?

Physician: Of course I like pets. But that's not the point.

Director: What is the point? We know what truths to grasp.

Physician: Yes, but we don't know what happens when we do.

Director: Didn't we just lay it all out?

Physician: Director, can't you be serious?

Director: Alright. I'll tell you the truth. Truth grasping is an adventure.

Physician: I believe that's so. But then do you know what else I want to know?

Director: Of course. You want to know if adventure is required for health.

Physician: Is it?

Director: Well, there's health... and then there's health.

49

Physician: Oh, don't do that. Let's just say a boring life can make us sick.

Director: Okay. A boring life can make us sick.

Physician: But we all have the power not to be bored.

Director: We do. We just gobble up those truths.

Physician: Now, I want you to tell me, exactly, how digesting truths frees us from boredom.

Director: When we take in truth, we can't help but change how we act.

Physician: And when we change how we act?

Director: Others react.

Physician: And when others react?

Director: Our circumstances change.

Physician: And change in circumstance makes for adventure?

Director: It's a chain reaction. Change brings change, and who knows where it leads?

Physician: That's scary for many.

Director: What's the alternative? Isn't it always less frightening when you're bored?

Physician: Yes, it is. And being bored can make you ill. But I wonder about the opposite. Can too much adventure make you sick?

Director: If it can, what's the best way to proceed?

Physician: Start out small and see how it goes.

Director: We should experiment carefully with change?

Physician: Yes, without a doubt. You might overwhelm yourself if you don't.

Director: What things should we change?

Physician: The things that have to do with boredom.

Director: So we might change what we have for dinner?

Physician: Why not?

Director: Change who we have as our friends?

Physician: Well, that's a more radical change.

Director: What if we just make one new friend?

Physician: That's good. But it should be a different kind of friend.

Director: Not like the ones we already have?

Physician: Yes, the friend should be something new.

Director: What's the 'something new'? This person holds new truths?

Physician: I think that would be best.

Director: But we can't take on these truths all at once, can we?

Physician: You're right. We might just start with one.

Director: And share one of our own?

Physician: An even trade, yes.

Director: How long do you think this can go on?

Physician: The exchange of new truths? Well, how many truths do you think someone can have?

Director: I don't know. But I know we all should at least have one.

Physician: And is that truth a truth about the world?

Director: It's a truth about us, a truth we find in our core.

Physician: And is this what makes us who we are, this truth about us?

Director: That and the other truths we hold.

Physician: Do we share this truth?

Director: Not so fast. Don't you think it takes great trust to share something like this?

Physician: Naturally.

Director: And once shared, we can never take it back?

Physician: If it's been fully shared? No, never.

Director: You raise an interesting point.

Physician: How so?

Director: When you say 'fully shared', you imply it's possible to share less of it than all.

Physician: What's interesting about that?

Director: We might engage in a sort of dance. Share a little here, then dance around. Share a little there, and dance away. And so on.

Physician: That might be fun.

Director: Yes, and is fun ever boring?

Physician: True fun? No. And I can tell you as a doctor that fun can be healthy.

Director: Then let's have some fun.

50

Physician: So dance!

Director: Here's the first step. It's a question. What happens when you get a taste of my core truth?

Physician: I don't know. What happens?

Director: You can't help but change.

Physician: Why?

Director: Do you really think you can learn something important and not change?

Physician: Ha, ha! So you believe your truth is important? Well, I think you have a point! So what's the next step?

Director: Next is a series of questions. How do I stop the dance from turning into a tease?

Physician: You share more.

Director: And if I don't share more?

Physician: You'll frustrate your friend.

Director: Why would this friend get frustrated? That can't be good for their health.

Physician: The friend gets frustrated because they want to know!

Director: And they think it's their right to know?

Physician: After enough time as a friend? Yes.

Director: That's where they're wrong. We never have a right to a friend's truth. The friend has to want to share.

Physician: But what if we figure it out on our own?

Director: What if?

Physician: Tell me. Do you think you've figured me out?

Director: I think I have much to learn.

Physician: Well, I know I haven't figured you out yet.

Director: What would you like to know?

Physician: You'd tell me? Just like that?

Director: Just like that. So what would you like to know?

Physician: What's the most important thing in the world to you?

Director: Didn't we just answer that?

Physician: Yes, but I want you to be specific.

Director: How can I be more specific than by saying it's love?

Physician: Love for what?

Director: All that's worth loving.

Physician: Is philosophy worth loving?

Director: Do you doubt it is?

Physician: I don't know. It's not something I love.

Director: What's something you love?

Physician: My friends.

Director: I love my friends, too.

Physician: Yes, but I want to know how that love compares to your love for philosophy.

Director: You mean, is one more important than the other?

Physician: Yes.

Director: Well, I think there's something of a mystery here.

Physician: Why?

Director: Because I'm not sure how to answer.

Physician: Tell me what you think.

Director: It'll help me bring it out if you answer a few questions.

Physician: What do you want to know?

Director: Are you my friend for the sake of furthering my philosophy?

Physician: That's something you should tell me.

Director: In order to tell you, we need to know — what is philosophy?

Physician: You're asking me? If I had to say, I suppose I'd say it's knowing the truth.

Director: Do you love knowing the truth?

Physician: Of course I do.

Director: So doesn't that make you something of a philosopher? As such, would you be ashamed to be known as someone who helps me know truth?

Physician: No, I wouldn't.

Director: Then tell me. This truth that you help me know, do we share it?

Physician: Yes, certainly.

Director: And is it possible that this sharing will make our friendship grow?

Physician: It's more than possible. Sharing will definitely make our friendship grow.

Director: So it's philosophy for the sake of friendship.

Physician: It is. Then are you saying friendship is the more important thing?

Director: I find that hard to say.

Physician: Why?

Director: Because true friendship contributes to something beyond itself.

Physician: Let me guess. It contributes its truth to philosophy.

Director: Yes. So then isn't it friendship for the sake of philosophy? Do you see the dilemma? I don't know what to say.

Physician: Director, you've painted yourself into a corner. There's no mystery here, no reason to be perplexed.

Director: Why not?

Physician: Because it's symbiosis! The relationship of friendship and philosophy is to the advantage of both!

Director: Well, I'm relieved! So let's conclude that the best friends are those who love each other — and love philosophy, too.

51

Physician: So you really have love in your core.

Director: And in your core, Physician?

Physician: Love.

Director: Then no wonder we make such excellent friends. But have we given ourselves away?

Physician: It's one thing to say you love. But it's another to show what that means.

Director: Maybe that's the dance. Showing what love means to all your friends.

Physician: I think that's true. But....

Director: But what?

Physician: Our friends aren't the same.

Director: Not the same as us?

Physician: No, I mean we don't share friends in common.

Director: So I don't love the friends you love?

Physician: And I don't love the friends you love, either.

Director: What's wrong with that?

Physician: Our friends are part of our core.

Director: So we can't fully share our core if we don't share friends?

Physician: Yes. Do you agree?

Director: Well.... I mean....

Physician: What's the problem?

Director: I know what you're saying, but I don't agree.

Physician: Why not?

Director: We don't have to think of friends as part of our core.

Physician: Then how should we think of them?

Director: As ships that dock with us for a time.

Physician: And then off they sail?

Director: Yes, until they come back. And some come back every single day.

Physician: Then what's the point?

Director: We all have more freedom this way.

Physician: I suppose. But I really don't like what you're saying. I like the idea of a friend being part of me.

Director: But then we have the problem you raised when it comes to sharing friends.

Physician: So what can we do?

Director: I'm not sure. But there's another problem with thinking this way.

Physician: What?

Director: What if a friend gets sick and loses their way?

Physician: Do you want to know if we share in the sickness and lose our way, too, because they're part of us?

Director: Well? What do you think?

Physician: We must keep to our way and avoid the sickness.

Director: So we cast our friend out of our heart and abandon them on the side of the road?

Physician: No, no, no — of course not. But what do you think we should do?

Director: We have to nurse our friend, and help keep them on their way.

52

Physician: So how do we nurse?

Director: You, a doctor, don't know how to nurse?

Physician: Let's pretend I don't know.

Director: Alright. A good nurse helps a patient take an interest in life.

Physician: How?

Director: By encouraging them to take up the fight.

Physician: And how does the nurse do that?

Director: By being a mirror.

Physician: What do you mean?

Director: The nurse shows the patient his or her intrinsically interesting self.

Physician: And then the patient wants to fight for that self?

Director: Yes. Don't you agree?

Physician: I do. And I believe that fight helps keep them on their way. But you know what my next question must be, don't you?

Director: You want to know what happens if the patient's self isn't interesting at all.

Physician: Well?

Director: What self isn't interesting?

Physician: The self that doesn't take an interest in others.

Director: You need to take an interest in order to be of interest?

Physician: Yes. Do you agree?

Director: I do. But, to be sure, if you're interesting, does that mean you have the potential to be healthy?

Physician: If you take a healthy interest in yourself and others? Yes, of course.

Director: What would it mean to take an unhealthy interest in yourself and others?

Physician: Maybe you're too interested?

Director: How could you be too interested?

Physician: You neglect other things.

Director: What things are there other than yourself and others?

Physician: You might neglect your business.

Director: Business? What business do you have other than with others and yourself?

Physician: Then maybe there's no such thing as unhealthy interest.

Director: Not even if it amounts to obsession?

Physician: Well, yes. Why didn't you say so in the first place? Obsession is unhealthy.

Director: What's the specific difference between interest and obsession?

Physician: Interest occupies your mind. Obsession obtrudes upon it.

Director: When your mind is occupied your mind is working?

Physician: Yes.

Director: What's the proper work of the mind?

Physician: Thinking.

Director: And we can't think when we're obsessed?

Physician: No, we can't.

Director: But does that mean we can't think our way through an obsession?

Physician: We can — if we get away.

Director: What do you mean?

Physician: We have to escape from the object of obsession or we won't be able to think.

Director: I can see how that might work with others. We need time away, and maybe permanently. But if we're obsessed with ourselves? How do we get away from ourselves?

Physician: We focus on external things. Things that demand our attention.

Director: But if things demand our attention, how do we have time to think?

Physician: We think when we're done with the external things.

Director: But then what stops us from obsessing again?

Physician: Maybe the external things gave us some perspective.

Director: Perspective is the enemy of obsession?

Physician: Yes, I think that's true.

Director: So if we have perspective we can think about ourselves in a healthy way?

Physician: Don't you agree?

Director: That sounds right to me. But what's there to think about when we think about ourselves?

Physician: What kind of person we are.

Director: What does that mean?

Physician: Oh, you know. Whether we're hypocrites, for instance.

Director: So this thinking about ourselves is a moral exercise?

Physician: I think it is.

Director: Hmm. And in this moral exercise we judge ourselves?

Physician: Yes.

Director: I don't know, Physician. But, in your view, is thinking about ourselves wholly a moral exercise, or is it also something else?

Physician: It's also something else.

Director: What?

Physician: I'm not sure. I just feel there should be something more.

Director: Well, can we think about the things we want?

Physician: Sure. But how much thinking does that require?

Director: Oh, I think it can take a fair amount, at times.

Physician: Times when our wants aren't clear?

Director: Don't you think there are times like that?

Physician: I do. But what else can we think when we think about ourselves?

Director: We can think about what we think.

Physician: Our opinions, you mean?

Director: Yes. And why not? Shouldn't we examine our opinions?

Physician: I think we should. What else?

Director: We can think about our actions, in the sense of trying to understand them.

Physician: What's to understand?

Director: Why we did them. How things worked out. What we can do in the future. Do you agree?

Physician: I agree.

Director: Can you think of anything else?

Physician: I can't.

53

Director: When we think about others, do we think about these same things?

Physician: I suppose we must. We think about what they want. We think about their opinions. And we think about their actions.

Director: And that should give us plenty to think about?

Physician: If we have many people to think about? Yes.

Director: And if we start to feel obsessed with any one of them?

Physician: We need to get away and think the obsession through.

Director: Tell me. What is it that causes us to become obsessed?

Physician: Well, we could be infatuated with someone's looks.

Director: True. What else?

Physician: I suppose there could be something fascinating in their personality.

Director: Fascinating in what sense?

Physician: They might say amazing things, do amazing things.

Director: Things we can't quite figure out?

Physician: Exactly. And then we just can't get enough.

Director: Let's flip things around. Would you like to cause obsession in others?

Physician: Ha! That's an interesting question. I'm not sure.

Director: Why not?

Physician: Because what good comes of it?

Director: It's flattering, isn't it?

Physician: I guess. But it might be a real pain.

Director: How so?

Physician: The obsessed would never leave you alone.

Director: And you like to be left alone?

Physician: Who doesn't?

Director: Someone who enjoys being the object of obsession.

Physician: I think that amounts to illness.

Director: Why?

Physician: There's no healthy relationship between the obsessed and the object of their obsession.

Director: But if the relationship were between someone who likes to think and the object of their thought?

Physician: Well, I suppose that might be healthier.

Director: What would make it fully healthy?

Physician: Both individuals thinking and being the object of the other's thought.

Director: Reciprocal thought is the ideal?

Physician: Yes.

Director: So if you think about someone but they don't think about you?

Physician: It's no good.

Director: I wonder. Is thinking the same as caring?

Physician: No, of course not.

Director: But if you care, you think?

Physician: You should.

Director: And that's why we say someone is 'thoughtful'? Because they think?

Physician: Yes.

Director: Is being thoughtful always good?

Physician: Maybe not always.

Director: When wouldn't it be?

Physician: When dealing with someone who treats you poorly.

Director: You don't need to think about how to treat them back?

Physician: Yes, you do. But it doesn't make sense to be 'thoughtful' with them.

Director: What makes sense?

Physician: Making the poor treatment stop.

Director: How can you do that?

Physician: For one? You can leave. But you can't torment yourself.

Director: What do you mean?

Physician: We sometimes feel like cowards when we leave.

Director: Why?

Physician: Because we imagine there was more we could have done.

Director: More to improve the situation?

Physician: Yes. We beat ourselves up over this.

Director: And do ourselves wrong?

Physician: Of course.

Director: And that's not healthy.

Physician: It's very unhealthy.

Director: Tell me now. Is it easy to leave a bad situation?

Physician: It's very difficult.

Director: So we might say it takes courage to leave.

Physician: You know, that's a very good point.

Director: And courage is healthy?

Physician: Very healthy.

Director: Are courage and cowardice matters of mental health?

Physician: It's funny. We don't usually think of it that way.

Director: How do we usually think of it?

Physician: As matters of character.

Director: And character is a matter of the body?

Physician: No, it's not.

Director: Is it a matter of society?

Physician: Of course not.

Director: So it's definitely not a matter of the planet.

Physician: You know it's not.

Director: Then what else can it be but a matter of the mind?

Physician: I have to agree.

Director: So how does it work? If we have a bad character, can we have mental health?

Physician: No.

Director: We need a good character for mental health?

Physician: I think we do. Don't you?

Director: I'm inclined to say yes. But let's talk about something other than courage and cowardice for a moment. What's another pair that's a matter of character?

Physician: Kindness and cruelty.

Director: Now, is there any doubt that if you're kind you can have mental health?

Physician: None.

Director: But not all the kind are mentally healthy?

Physician: True. I know some mentally ill people who are very kind.

Director: Too kind at times?

Physician: Yes.

Director: Is it the same with courage?

Physician: I'm not sure you can be too courageous.

Director: Why not?

Physician: Courage is always good.

Director: But we can be foolhardy at times?

Physician: Yes, recklessly bold or rash — which isn't courage.

Director: Is there an analogue when it comes to being kind?

Physician: Being a fool.

Director: Do foolhardiness and foolishness compromise character?

Physician: They do. And they weaken our mental health.

54

Director: Now let's turn to cruelty. Does cruelty make for bad character?

Physician: I want to say yes, but I'm not sure that's always so.

Director: Why?

Physician: Haven't you ever heard the saying 'cruel to be kind'?

Director: I have.

Physician: Well, it means you can be cruel and still be of good character.

Director: Which means you might be of sound mental health.

Physician: Yes, but only when the cruelty truly amounts to kindness.

Director: Only? Are you sure?

Physician: When else is it good to be cruel?

Director: What if you're cruel to the cruel?

Physician: That makes me uneasy.

Director: How would you rather treat the cruel?

Physician: I'd rather deal with them effectively, but with....

Director: But with a kind heart?

Physician: No. But with no unnecessary cruelty.

Director: So it's only the necessary cruelty you like?

Physician: I don't like it. Liking it can make your character bad.

Director: Which would make you at least somewhat mentally ill?

Physician: Yes. But I have some trouble here.

Director: What trouble?

Physician: It sometimes seems to me that people can be cruel but perfectly sane.

Director: But sanity and mental health are two different things.

Physician: Tell me how so.

Director: What is sanity?

Physician: Being able to think and behave in a normal manner.

Director: And if cruelty is the norm?

Physician: I suppose the cruel one is sane.

Director: Now what about kindness? Is kindness the norm?

Physician: Hardly.

Director: So the kind are insane?

Physician: Ha, ha! They might be. But that doesn't prevent them from being healthy, as far as I'm concerned.

Director: Now tell me. Are the kind and cruel aware of their own states of health?

Physician: I suppose they must be, at some level.

Director: Suppose someone who's cruel gets to know someone who's kind. And the cruel one realizes the kind one is healthy. What will the cruel one want to do?

Physician: Learn to be kind?

Director: Really?

Physician: Learn... or attack.

Director: And if attacked, what should the kind one do?

Physician: Fight back.

Director: Now something you said comes back to me. Didn't you suggest we can enjoy a good fight?

Physician: I did. But I'd rather prevent the fight if I can.

Director: How would you do that?

Physician: I'd deter through strength.

Director: And if that doesn't work?

Physician: I don't know. Do you know of any other way?

Director: Hmm. I do know of an old way. But it's one that rarely works.

Physician: Anything is worth a try. So what's this way? What does it involve?

Director: Words.

Physician: Words? Ha, ha. Who speaks these words?

Director: Priestesses and priests.

Physician: And what do they say?

Director: Things to make the cruel ones feel sick.

Physician: How?

Director: By playing on their conscience.

Physician: Ha! And if the cruel have no conscience, and they decide to attack?

Director: Then we should feel good — in meeting their force with force.

55

Physician: Mental force or bodily force?

Director: Well, if we're attacked with mental force, how should we respond?

Physician: With mental force.

Director: And if we're attacked with bodily force?

Physician: We respond with bodily force — because those who attack with bodily force only understand similar force.

Director: And those who attack with mental force? What do they understand?

Physician: It's an interesting question. They understand both.

Director: So why limit ourselves to mental force with them?

Physician: Society expects that we use proportional force.

Director: Which is the greater force? The mental or the physical?

Physician: Yes, I know what you mean. Mental attacks can be more cruel than physical attacks.

Director: But we can still only fight them off with mental force.

Physician: Yes.

Director: Hmm. Suppose we're under mental attack, but we're not strong enough to resist appropriately. What do we do?

Physician: This, I think, is where many a tragedy is made.

Director: Oh?

Physician: The person under attack snaps and fights back physically.

Director: And why does that make for tragedy?

Physician: Because he or she will be blamed and punished for resorting to physical force.

Director: What other choice is there for the one under overwhelming mental attack?

Physician: They can go away and live to fight another day.

Director: Because while away they can build their mental strength?

Physician: Yes, so long as they know to keep away from the mentally cruel.

Director: Why wouldn't they keep away?

Physician: They might gravitate toward what they know.

Director: Really? Then they should learn to know new things.

Physician: Ah, you make it sound so easy.

Director: I'm not saying coming to know is easy. If all you know is sickness, health can be hard to learn.

Physician: Yes, and the healthy might be prejudiced against you.

Director: Why?

Physician: Because you'll seem strange to them as you learn.

Director: Because you're not simply healthy like them?

Physician: Yes. And because you're not quite sick, either.

Director: And what's the goal? To be healthy like them? To become like them?

Physician: No. But, you know, we're not just talking about sickness and health.

Director: What are we talking about?

Physician: The fact that someone once under attack can never be like those who were never under attack.

Director: So what's the goal?

Physician: Your goal is to become healthy, yes. But healthy in your own way.

Director: Then there are different kinds of health?

Physician: No, health is health. But how we achieve it varies.

Director: Do we achieve it when we're on our true way in life?

Physician: That's a very good question. And the answer is an emphatic yes!

Director: So finding our way is the key.

Physician: No doubt.

Director: But can we find our way if we're not healthy? I mean, is it health that allows us to find our way?

Physician: Is health required for health? Is that what you're asking? Well, I think you need some health in order to get more.

Director: What's your way, Physician?

Physician: It's not so easy to say. A way can be winding and not be as simple as we'd like. In life there are many twists and turns.

Director: Agreed. But at a basic level, how do you achieve your greater health?

Physician: I achieve it through healing.

Director: Then how fortunate you've got your new role.

Physician: Yes. But I have to tell you. I sometimes worry I won't heal as much in this role as I've healed in my practice.

Director: Well, what if you're right? You heal less. But what if you feel healthier nonetheless?

Physician: Then I'm wrong about what makes me healthy.

Director: You're really open to the possibility you might be wrong?

Physician: I like to think I am. It's difficult, but you have to be honest with yourself.

Director: Yes, but what about guilt?

Physician: Will I feel guilty if I don't heal at least as much as I have up until now? The answer is almost certainly yes.

Director: Is guilt healthy?

Physician: Not if it makes you stop doing what brings you health.

Director: But you have an ally in the fight against guilt, don't you?

Physician: Who, you?

Director: Yes, but I was thinking of something else.

Physician: What?

Director: Happiness.

Physician: Ah, an excellent point.

56

Director: Health and happiness together can overcome guilt.

Physician: I believe it's true. But we're always in danger of getting confused.

Director: Are we? How so?

Physician: When we speak of health, I can't always tell if we're talking about physical or mental health.

Director: But the two are so closely related.

Physician: All the more reason to distinguish more clearly!

Director: Okay. So let's observe that it's hard to pursue happiness without mental health.

Physician: But it's also hard to pursue happiness without physical health!

Director: It seems I'm at a loss.

Physician: Oh, you're not even trying.

Director: What can physical health help us with?

Physician: Mental health.

Director: And mental health can help us with happiness?

Physician: Yes.

Director: But what else can mental health help us with? Is it only happiness?

Physician: No, mental health can help us with physical health.

Director: And physical health can help us with happiness?

Physician: Yes. But we're going in circles. This is all hopelessly intertwined.

Director: I wouldn't say 'hopelessly'. Health, generally speaking, helps us with happiness.

Physician: And happiness helps us with health?

Director: Do you doubt it does? But maybe we should forget about happiness and keep our focus on health.

Physician: We'll just assume happiness will come?

Director: Isn't that what most people do?

Physician: Yes, but we're not most people.

Director: Then where do we put happiness? With physical or mental health?

Physician: I can't believe you're asking.

Director: Because the answer is so obvious?

Physician: Yes! Happiness is part of mental health.

Director: So be it. Except....

Physician: What now?

Director: What about those who suffer from depression?

Physician: What about them?

Director: They're not happy, are they?

Physician: They're the opposite of happy.

Director: And this is a mental illness?

Physician: Why do you have to ask?

Director: Because there's some reason to think it's a physical illness. After all, we said depression can affect the body. And don't we treat it with medicine, a physical means?

Physician: Yes, but we also treat depression with talk.

Director: But can't we call talk physical? We spoke of this, you know.

Physician: Yes, I know. What do you think?

Director: Let's say for now that depression is part physical and part mental.

Physician: That's fine with me.

Director: So what of its opposite?

Physician: Happiness? Part physical and part mental?

Director: Is it?

Physician: I suppose we have to say it is.

Director: Then let's say it.

Physician: Alright. But a crazy thought just occurred to me.

Director: Better get it out fast before it sets.

Physician: What about societal happiness? Is it, too, part physical and part mental?

Director: Well, what makes up society?

Physician: People.

Director: And we're sure people's happiness is part physical and part mental?

Physician: Pretty sure.

Director: Then we're pretty sure society's happiness is part physical and part mental.

Physician: But what does that mean?

Director: Look at it this way. If the people are starving, is society in a good way?

Physician: Of course not.

Director: And if the people are anxious, is society doing well?

Physician: No.

Director: Starvation is of the body and anxiety is of the mind?

Physician: Yes.

Director: Can starvation affect the mind?

Physician: Certainly.

Director: And can anxiety affect the body?

Physician: Without a doubt.

Director: Then things aren't so simple for society, either, my friend.

57

Physician: But it's simple for the planet.

Director: What do you mean?

Physician: There's no 'mental' for the planet. It's all physical.

Director: And does that 'physical' exist all for us or also for itself?

Physician: The planet can't exist for itself — because it hasn't got a self!

Director: Then the planet exists solely for us?

Physician: Yes, for all forms of life.

Director: Our physical and mental parts both?

Physician: Without the planet, neither our physical nor mental parts would exist.

Director: If that's true, then we need a healthy relationship between the planet and ourselves.

Physician: Certainly.

Director: Just as we need a healthy relationship between society and ourselves?

Physician: No doubt.

Director: Just as we need a healthy relationship between ourselves and others?

Physician: Yes.

Director: Then I wonder what you think about this. Do we need a healthy relationship with ourselves?

Physician: You mean, you with yourself and me with myself?

Director: That's what I mean.

Physician: We definitely need that.

Director: Now, there are always at least two parts to a relationship. Do you agree?

Physician: I do.

Director: What parts are we talking about when it comes to a relationship with ourselves?

Physician: The heart and the mind.

Director: Interesting. We haven't spoken about having a healthy heart. But let me say this. To have a good relationship, both parts to it must be mostly healthy, no?

Physician: Yes, both must be mostly healthy or the relationship will fail.

Director: What does it take to have a healthy heart?

Physician: Listening. You have to listen to your heart.

Director: Because the heart is always right?

Physician: Of course.

Director: And it's the mind that listens?

Physician: Yes.

Director: But doesn't the mind listen to itself?

Physician: I suppose.

Director: So why can't the heart listen to itself, too?

Physician: Oh, I don't know. Let's say it can.

Director: Yes, and let's say the heart can also listen to the mind. Do you object?

Physician: No, I think that's fine.

Director: So we have two parts of us listening to themselves and each other.

Physician: And that's healthy, depending on what they say.

Director: That makes me wonder. We said the heart is always right. But what if the heart is poisoned? That happens, doesn't it?

Physician: Yes, it certainly happens.

Director: Should we listen to a poisoned heart?

Physician: We should try to draw the poison off before we listen.

Director: How do we do that?

Physician: We reason with our heart.

Director: The heart reasons?

Physician: No. I mean, our mind speaks reason to the heart.

Director: Oh. Is that an easy thing to do?

Physician: I don't think there's anything harder.

Director: Because the heart won't listen?

Physician: Because the heart thinks it's right.

Director: But deep down inside it knows it's wrong, it knows the poison worked its harm?

Physician: That's what I like to believe.

Director: So we have to reason our way deep down inside — and do what?

Physician: Encourage the true heart to spit out the poison.

Director: And if it does?

Physician: The heart can have a healthy relationship with the mind.

Director: But suppose there's so much poison nothing can be done.

Physician: That person will always be sick.

Director: Will the heart eventually poison the mind?

Physician: All but certainly.

Director: So the person becomes one great big ball of poison?

Physician: Yes, but as a healer I have to believe there's some hope.

Director: But you said this person will always be sick.

Physician: There are varying degrees of sickness.

Director: You'd spend your precious healing time on those who, at best, show just a little improvement?

Physician: You can learn a lot from people like that.

Director: What can you learn?

Physician: How a touch of true heart can go a long way.

Director: The touch being theirs. But what about you and your true heart?

Physician: Every true healer puts their heart into the work.

Director: So a requirement for healers is to have a pure heart. Or can you heal with a heart full of poison?

Physician: If your heart were full of poison, you wouldn't want to heal. And yes, you need a pure heart — or one that's pure enough, since no one's heart is perfectly pure.

Director: Does the act of healing increase the purity of a more or less pure heart?

Physician: That's an excellent question. And the answer is yes.

Director: And the more you heal, the more you'll want to heal?

Physician: That's the dynamic.

Director: Now I wonder about this. Can you have a wonderfully pure heart — and not want to heal?

Physician: Why wouldn't you want to heal?

Director: I don't know. What do you think?

Physician: I think the answer is no. Because if you have an opportunity to help heal a heart or mind, and turn it down, that darkens your heart a shade.

Director: And if you turn down opportunities all the time, eventually your heart becomes black?

Physician: I'm afraid it's true.

Director: How do we know when we have an opportunity?

Physician: We have to know what's wrong, or at least have an idea.

Director: How do we know what's wrong?

Physician: We talk.

Director: Philosophers talk.

Physician: Yes, and I believe they often figure out what's wrong.

Director: But knowing what's wrong and helping are two different things.

Physician: Sometimes telling another what's wrong is help enough.

Director: I agree. But sometimes it's not. What, if anything, can we do then?

Physician: We can give them an answer.

Director: A way to respond to what's wrong?

Physician: Exactly.

Director: To be clear, you're saying we tell them what to do?

Physician: Oh, I know. That's a risky business. But what other choice do we have?

Director: Hmm. Wouldn't we have to know them very well before telling them what to do?

Physician: Yes, very.

Director: And that takes time?

Physician: A great amount of it.

Director: But do we always have that time? I mean, don't we at times have to perform triage?

Physician: You know, that's a good point.

Director: What happens when we do?

Physician: We weigh what we know, say what we can — and then we move on.

59

Director: Can we triage society?

Physician: When it's sick? Yes, I think we can.

Director: How do we do that?

Physician: We start with the leaders.

Director: The leaders? But won't they be hardest to deal with?

Physician: Often times? Yes. But why do you say that?

Director: Because leaders can be self-important.

Physician: Ha, ha. That's true.

Director: Tell me why it's difficult to heal the self-important.

Physician: Because they won't listen to us.

Director: And isn't there something else? Something before it's time for them to listen?

Physician: They won't let us in to see what we need to see.

Director: So maybe it's better to find leaders who aren't self-important and start with them?

Physician: Yes, they're the ones we should approach.

Director: And what will we say when we approach? 'You're sick and need our help'?

Physician: Of course not.

Director: So what do we do?

Physician: We see if we can engage their interest.

Director: How might we do that?

Physician: We can talk about what they care about.

Director: And see if they'll let us in.

Physician: Right. And if they do, we'll try to figure out what their problem is.

Director: And so on, and so on — until they have their answer?

Physician: Yes.

Director: What do we do then? Just up and move along?

Physician: Well, we might spend more time with leaders than we would with others.

Director: Why?

Physician: To ensure they do what they must in order to heal.

Director: And if they won't?

Physician: Then the answer lies in the future.

Director: The future leaders?

Physician: Yes, the young. They might be society's cure.

Director: What do we say to them?

Physician: We show them how and why society is sick.

Director: So they'll figure out what they must do?

Physician: Yes.

Director: But do we tell them about the self-important?

Physician: Of course we do.

Director: What happens if word gets back to the self-important that we're 'corrupting the youth' this way?

Physician: What do you think happens?

Director: They'll attack.

Physician: They'll attack us?

Director: Yes. Why? Do you think they'd attack the young?

Physician: They'll attack whoever stands opposed to what they want.

Director: And what do they want?

Physician: To let their illness grow.

Director: Oh, but who really wants an illness to grow?

Physician: If the illness is an exaggerated sense of self?

Director: Well, you may have a point. But what can we do?

Physician: All we can do is encourage the young and let them fight their fight.

Director: While we stand aside?

Physician: No! We hardly stand aside. We go on healing as many in the society as we can. That's our fight.

Director: And will the healed join in the effort?

Physician: Of course they will — because part of being healed is understanding what's at stake.

60

Director: So where will you start your fight?

Physician: I suppose I should start at my school.

Director: Why do you sound doubtful?

Physician: Because it might turn out to be an actual fight.

Director: When you start a fight, isn't that what you should expect? And here I was thinking you were ready to take on society.

Physician: I worry about my students.

Director: Why?

Physician: Because they need a place to learn in peace.

Director: What will they learn?

Physician: How to heal.

Director: How to heal without a fight?

Physician: Well....

Director: Did you think it was an accident we talked about kung fu?

Physician: I thought you were trying to lighten things up.

Director: That's true. I was. But I was also making a point.

Physician: The point that fighting isn't serious?

Director: Oh, it's serious alright. And that's why fighters need a little comic relief.

Physician: The comedy keeps them healthy?

Director: It keeps them from getting sick of fighting, yes.

Physician: I suppose that's true. If you're too serious about anything you grow sick.

Director: Even if you're too serious about healing?

Physician: Even so.

Director: When do things lighten up when it comes to health?

Physician: When you meet with success.

Director: You mean, when someone is healed?

Physician: Yes.

Director: And if that someone stays sick?

Physician: That's not so comic.

Director: It's more tragic?

Physician: Of course.

Director: Then would you only attempt to heal those who seem to have a good chance of being healed?

Physician: No! I always try to heal them all.

Director: But what about triage?

Physician: Triage doesn't mean you only take the easy cases.

Director: But you do give up on those without hope?

Physician: Well, if forced to, yes.

Director: And there's nothing light hearted in that.

Physician: Absolutely nothing.

Director: Tell me. Do you ever think of yourself in a comic way?

Physician: Do you?

Director: Think of myself? Yes, from time to time.

Physician: You think I should, too?

Director: Don't you think it's healthier that way?

Physician: Not if it leads to buffoonery.

Director: Physician, if you were someone who could be a buffoon, I'd never have said the things I've said to you today.

Physician: Then you're talking about a light touch of comedy?

Director: The lightest of touches, my friend. And that's enough.

61

Physician: Yes, but we're talking about ourselves. What about our patients? Is the lightest touch of comedy all it takes with them?

Director: Yes and no.

Physician: Why do you say that?

Director: Because sometimes they need a fair amount of the comic, but we can't give it to them all at once.

Physician: Why not?

Director: Don't patients rightly expect their healers will be serious in the healing?

Physician: Of course.

Director: Then we can see why healers can only use a light touch of comedy here and there — never too much.

Physician: But over time it all adds up?

Director: Yes.

Physician: How do we know when comedy is required?

Director: We look for an overdose.

Physician: Of what?

Director: Seriousness.

Physician: What does that look like?

Director: Oh, I think you'll be able to tell.

Physician: But what about the opposite?

Director: A comic overdose? Have you ever seen one?

Physician: I've seen people who joke all the time. They strike me as sad inside.

Director: If they're sad, comedy isn't performing its function.

Physician: Which is?

Director: To make the spirit light.

Physician: Does that mean the function of seriousness is to make the spirit heavy?

Director: I think that follows, don't you? So what should a spirit be?

Physician: I knew you'd put that question to me. If I give you my answer, will you give me yours?

Director: I will.

Physician: A spirit should be between heavy and light. Otherwise, the spirit might be too comic and unable to take anything seriously. Or the spirit might be too serious and unable to take anything lightly.

Director: So if someone takes nothing, absolutely nothing seriously, we know there's something wrong.

Physician: We do.

Director: And if someone takes nothing, absolutely nothing lightly, we also know there's something wrong.

Physician: We certainly do.

Director: Would it be fair to say the former needs a touch of the serious, and the latter needs a touch of the comic?

Physician: It would be more than fair.

Director: So, given all this, health amounts to what?

Physician: Taking things seriously when you must, and taking things lightly when you can.

Director: But why not take things seriously when we can, and lightly when we must?

Physician: I suppose it depends on what you expect to find in the world.

Director: That's very profound.

Physician: Oh, you're just teasing. You want to suggest there isn't much to take seriously in life.

Director: If you long for the serious, the things worth taking seriously — wouldn't you take anything seriously that you can? And wouldn't all the comedy seem like an unfortunate must?

Physician: That might be true.

Director: But if you long for the comic, and so on and so on — it's the opposite truth, yes?

Physician: I think it is.

62

Director: Well, that's enough of that. What shall we talk about now?

Physician: The answer you never gave — what a spirit should be. I said it should be between heavy and light.

Director: Yes, you did.

Physician: What do you say?

Director: I say a spirit should be both heavy and light at once.

Physician: How is that possible?

Director: It's heavy in regard to some things, and light in regard to others.

Physician: At the same time?

Director: Yes, or at least as close to 'at the same time' as two things can be. Suppose you encounter two people, and one is too heavy and one is too light. What do you do?

Physician: I don't know.

Director: You act appropriately. You're somewhat heavy with the light one and somewhat light with the heavy.

Physician: And what does that accomplish?

Director: It soothes.

Physician: Ha! It soothes?

Director: If it's done right? Yes, of course.

Physician: What comes of the soothing?

Director: At best, those soothed learn how they can sooth themselves.

Physician: And soothing heals?

Director: Soothing heals.

Physician: But what if you're being 'somewhat' heavy or light with someone, and it's not enough?

Director: Then sterner means might be required.

Physician: Sterner means? Ha, ha. I can see how to be stern with someone who's too light. You just become more serious. But how can you be stern with someone who's too heavy?

Director: You employ a barb that only he or she can feel.

Physician: What kind of barb?

Director: Say the serious one is talking to others about serious things. You step in lightly and joke in a gentle, friendly way about whatever they're talking about.

Physician: And that's it?

Director: Not quite. When you joke, you have to show you have a firm grip on the topics in question. You make clear that if you wanted to be serious, you could. The serious one has to know this, has to feel it.

Physician: Feel that the serious topics admit of some levity?

Director: Yes. That's the barb. And if you performed well, the serious one might take it.

Physician: But you'd have to be an expert in the subjects discussed.

Director: I don't know about being an expert. You just have to know enough.

Physician: You have to be able to get to the heart of the matter?

Director: Yes.

Physician: And when you do, the overly serious one will see that he or she needs to lighten up, if only a touch?

Director: If all goes well? That's the revelation.

Physician: This all sounds like it takes a great deal of tact.

Director: It does. Especially because you don't want to go too far.

Physician: You just want to lighten things up the tiniest bit?

Director: Don't you think that makes for all the difference in the world?

Physician: I do. But now I wonder. Do you think health can be taken too seriously?

Director: Of course. What do we call that? Hypochondria?

Physician: No, not quite. That has to do with anxiety about health.

Director: You think the anxious don't take things seriously?

Physician: Yes, but you can take things too seriously and not be anxious.

Director: Then I don't know what the word is for taking health too seriously.

Physician: I don't either. But it's a real condition.

Director: Who will listen to us if we tell them not to be overly serious about health?

Physician: I don't know. People who are blessed with very good health?

Director: That might be. But certainly not people in very poor health?

Physician: They have reason to take their health very seriously.

Director: What happens if they don't take it seriously?

Physician: Then they're not going to get better.

Director: Yes, but say they take their health just a little bit lightly, and take all the necessary steps to get better.

Physician: They may well get better. And it's better to get better this way.

63

Director: Better because they've left room for a touch of the comic.

Physician: Right.

Director: But what if someone leaves too much room?

Physician: They're not serious enough about the necessary steps? Then something is wrong.

Director: Something in the mind?

Physician: Yes.

Director: Do you think it's a matter of attitude?

Physician: In many cases, it is. But why do you ask?

Director: I've heard people say 'attitude is everything'.

Physician: And so it is.

Director: So is attitude adjustment the business of healers?

Physician: Well, yes. To some degree.

Director: Why only to some degree?

Physician: Because attitude adjustment is a very difficult thing.

Director: What's the worst attitude you've encountered?

Physician: The worst? I've had patients who spurned the importance of health.

Director: Really? There's obviously something wrong when someone spurns the importance of health. So what did you tell them it is?

Physician: What do you mean?

Director: The importance of health. What did you tell them?

Physician: That nothing is more important.

Director: And they didn't believe you?

Physician: No, I can't say they did.

Director: That's a shame, because isn't health more important now than ever?

Physician: That's what I believe. But why do you say that?

Director: There's more we can do about it now.

Physician: You mean because medical sciences have advanced? I agree. And there's every indication they'll keep on advancing.

Director: How far do you think they'll go?

Physician: Barring cataclysms or profound and negative changes of heart? We'll one day create healthy human beings.

Director: From birth?

Physician: How else?

Director: And the goal will be perfect health?

Physician: Of course.

Director: But what about the advantage of sickness? I mean, what about insight, perspective, true vision? Or do we just forget what we said about those things?

Physician: No, we shouldn't forget. But I feel torn.

Director: How so?

Physician: I want perfect health and the advantages of sickness both.

Director: Is there a way to have both?

Physician: Maybe one day, when we have perfect health, we can create simulations that show the points of view of every sort of sickness.

Director: We'll get perspective on the cheap?

Physician: Well....

Director: And will we really trust in simulations?

Physician: Why wouldn't we?

Director: Because how can we ever know if a simulation accurately represents the real?

Physician: We can experiment.

Director: On whom? Healthy people? I don't know, Physician. Let's forget about experiments for now. And let's say the simulations are real enough that we can learn from them. What's their purpose? What do they help us do?

Physician: They help us find our way.

Director: And when we find our way, we have to choose it, don't we?

Physician: What do you mean by 'choose'?

Director: Make it our own. Or do you think finding the way is enough?

Physician: No, I like the idea of choosing it once it's found.

Director: Then tell me. Is choosing our way a serious thing?

Physician: There's nothing more serious.

Director: So maybe a touch of the light is appropriate here?

Physician: What kind of touch?

Director: Something unnecessary.

Physician: What do you have in mind?

Director: Laughter.

Physician: You'd laugh at our choice of way?

Director: Why not? Even if we laugh we still have to choose, and choice is still a very serious thing.

Physician: But you're not talking about gales of laughter, are you?

Director: No, I'm talking about a single, powerful 'ha!'

Physician: Would you say we can't be fully healthy if we never laugh that laugh?

Director: I would. But then we have a difficulty.

Physician: What difficulty?

Director: We're saying laughter is unnecessary and necessary both.

Physician: Then we should laugh at our need for laughter.

Director: Why not laugh at all of necessity?

Physician: So long as we do what's necessary? Why not?

Director: Tell me, Physician. Is necessity something safe?

Physician: I think it often involves danger.

Director: Then we'll laugh at danger?

Physician: If we do, people will think there's something wrong with us.

Director: I thought we were still talking about our single, powerful 'ha!' But really, is courage somehow wrong?

Physician: Laughter and courage are different things.

Director: Yes, but not as different as some might think. But even if they're as different as can be, do you agree both are necessary for health?

Physician: I do.

Director: So they should figure into our simulations?

Physician: But our simulations were of every possible sickness.

Director: Then maybe we need to see the effect of the absence of courage and laughter.

Physician: I agree.

Director: Good. Now, who makes the simulations?

Physician: We do.

Director: Do we make them, or do we make the computers that make them?

Physician: Well, of course — we make the computers and tell them to show us the various points of view.

Director: Of every possible sickness?

Physician: Yes. But now that we're at it, let's include every possible health.

Director: I thought we said health is health.

Physician: We're looking for the ways to health.

Director: Does it take courage to choose our way among all the potential ways to health?

Physician: Of course it does.

Director: Even if the computer finds the way for us?

Physician: We still have to have the courage to walk our way.

Director: Yes, but what about the computer? Does it need courage?

Physician: To find our way? Of course not. Computers can't have courage. They can't have laughter, either.

Director: So they can never be healthy in our sense?

Physician: No, they can't.

64

Director: But wouldn't it be better if they could be healthy that way?

Physician: Ha, ha. Sure, Director. So tell me, if you could give a computer one, either laughter or courage, which would it be?

Director: I'd choose laughter, a sense of humor.

Physician: Why?

Director: Because a true sense of humor can lead to courage.

Physician: But can't true courage lead to humor?

Director: A very good question. Maybe we'd better say what courage and humor are.

Physician: It's obvious that courage is facing your fear. But what would you say about humor?

Director: Humor is taking lightly what should be taken lightly.

Physician: And how does courage develop from that?

Director: If you know what to take lightly, you can learn what to take seriously. And knowing that is half the battle in being brave.

Physician: By learning to take seriously, do you mean learning what to fear?

Director: Yes.

Physician: But we all know what we fear!

Director: But do we all fear the right things?

Physician: And that's what courage is? Fearing the right things?

Director: And facing that fear, yes.

Physician: Well, you may have a point. Though you can't tell me it doesn't take courage to face even an irrational fear.

Director: Okay. But what about courage leading to humor?

Physician: If you know what to fear, what to take seriously, that's half the battle in having humor.

Director: Because you can learn what to take lightly?

Physician: Yes. What do you think?

Director: It appears to work both ways, courage to humor and humor to courage. So our chances of knowing how to take things in general seem very good, if we start with one or the other.

Physician: And how will computers start with one or the other?

Director: I don't know.

Physician: Neither do I. But they'd have to know on their own.

Director: What do you mean by that?

Physician: They'd have to know without being told.

Director: They'd figure it out themselves?

Physician: Yes, just like humans do.

Director: But do we know how humans do this?

Physician: No, we don't. It's a big question. One we can leave to the machines.

Director: Do you really mean that?

Physician: What if I do? If they can figure out how we know on our own, they can teach themselves to know on their own, as well.

Director: And then we can learn about ourselves from them?

Physician: Exactly.

Director: I see. And will these knowing computers have health?

Physician: Well, what makes a machine healthy?

Director: Doing its work well.

Physician: I think that's true.

Director: Is that different from what makes a human healthy?

Physician: Yes, of course.

Director: But is it? Can't we speak of our 'work' in a very broad sense?

Physician: We can. But our work is still different than the work of machines.

Director: How is it different?

Physician: Oh, you can't be serious.

Director: But I am. Perhaps it's better to ask where the work comes from.

Physician: The work of the machine is defined by humans.

Director: And the work of humans?

Physician: They define that themselves.

Director: And if the machine comes to define its own work?

Physician: Are you asking if it would be human?

Director: Well?

Physician: No, of course not.

Director: What would make it human?

Physician: You're asking seriously?

Director: Maybe I'm asking playfully. But I'm asking nonetheless.

65

Physician: You really think it's possible to make machines human?

Director: Well, if they can develop a sense of humor.... But we're sure humans have humor?

Physician: Of course we are.

Director: You can't be human without humor?

Physician: Not a healthy human, anyway. But let's talk about something else.

Director: You've had enough? But we were just getting started.

Physician: The truth is, I don't care about machines. And I certainly don't care about their human-like health.

Director: What do you care about?

Physician: Human health.

Director: I care about human health. I care about my health and the health of my friends.

Physician: Is that really all you care about?

Director: Shouldn't it be?

Physician: No! You should care about everyone's health.

Director: Why?

Physician: Because we want to make the world a better place!

Director: If everyone cared for themselves and their friends, wouldn't it be a better place?

Physician: Yes, but you're not 'everyone'.

Director: Who am I?

Physician: Someone who cares about health in a larger sense.

Director: But isn't it hard enough to care for our own?

Physician: And 'our own' is us and our friends?

Director: What else would you have it be?

Physician: Tell me. How do you choose your friends?

Director: Like a robot would.

Physician: Now you're just teasing again.

Director: No, really. How would a robot choose its friends?

Physician: I suppose it would choose the most healthy it could find.

Director: Is there anything wrong with that?

Physician: But what about the sick?

Director: You're worried we're being unfair to them, we're leaving them out?

Physician: Yes.

Director: Maybe we need to clear something up. What kind of sickness and health are we talking about?

Physician: You tell me.

Director: The sickness and health of character. Does that make a difference to how you feel?

Physician: Well, yes. It does.

Director: Will you make friends with those of unhealthy character?

Physician: Why would I?

Director: I thought you might want to heal them.

Physician: You don't have to be friends in order to heal.

Director: But those you heal might become your friends?

Physician: I suppose that's possible.

Director: But it would be easier to find healthy friends ready made.

Physician: I don't know that I'd say it's easy to find healthy friends.

Director: You make a good point. Though, in fairness, I said 'easier'.

Physician: Why is it easier?

Director: Are you asking in earnest? I think you know the answer.

Physician: I want to know what you think.

Director: Alright. It's easier because character isn't easily changed. Unless, of course, we're talking about the character of a machine. And even then....

Physician: Oh, why did you have to go back to that?

Director: Because this is the age we're in.

66

Physician: Then what should we do? Make healthy machines, and let them be the models for our human friends?

Director: I know that's not what you think we should do.

Physician: How do you know?

Director: Because I know the healthy, organic human is the only model for you.

Physician: Well, you're right.

Director: So if anything is modeled on anything else, it's machines on our healthy friends?

Physician: Yes, but then we'd better be very sure what 'healthy' is.

Director: My, have I ever heard you put 'healthy' in quotes?

Physician: Do you think that's bad?

Director: I think it's a sign of perspective.

Physician: What perspective?

Director: You know that 'healthy' isn't always healthy.

Physician: It's no surprise that what some people call 'healthy' isn't healthy at all.

Director: How do you know what's healthy, truly healthy?

Physician: Health is true when it lets you flourish.

Director: Like a plant?

Physician: Yes. And don't they say 'bloom where you're planted'?

Director: They do. But that doesn't mean they're right.

Physician: Would you rather wither where you're planted?

Director: I'd rather find the right place to set down my roots.

Physician: And how do you do that?

Director: I look for true friends.

Physician: And plant yourself with them?

Director: Do you have a better idea?

Physician: I don't.

Director: Then plant yourself with your true friends.

Physician: But by 'friends' you mean many things? Like friends and family both?

Director: I'm sorry you have to put 'friends' in quotes. But yes, 'friend' can mean many things.

Physician: Then there's nothing healthier than planting yourself with friends.

Director: And once we have, what do we have to do?

Physician: Maintain the friendships.

Director: How?

Physician: Through making an effort to understand.

Director: Ah.

Physician: What is it?

Director: I think that's exactly what we do.

Physician: No doubt. It's healthy to understand. And if it's healthy to understand, it's healthy to allow yourself to be understood.

Director: By just anyone?

Physician: No, of course not. We're talking about our friends.

Director: Is that our definition of friendship? Friends understand each other?

Physician: In a healthy friendship, yes.

Director: So if there's mutual understanding, we have a friend.

Physician: Well, I don't know.

Director: Why not?

Physician: You can have mutual understanding with an enemy.

Director: Is that understanding healthy?

Physician: I want to say all understanding is healthy. I mean, suppose you have this enemy and neither of you understands the other. Is that good? Might that not lead to unwanted conflict?

Director: So understanding, no matter of what, is healthy?

Physician: That's what I believe.

Director: Then what's the difference between an enemy and a friend?

Physician: With a friend you want to put down roots. With an enemy you want to get away.

Director: Get away from something you understand.

Physician: Right.

Director: So some things we understand are good, and some are bad?

Physician: Of course.

Director: And, to be sure. The good are healthy to be with.

Physician: Yes.

Director: And the bad are unhealthy to be with.

Physician: They are.

Director: Now here's what I wonder. Isn't your mission to heal the unhealthy, heal the sick?

Physician: Well, yes, it is.

Director: Then shouldn't you try to heal your enemies when they're sick?

Physician: I suppose you have a point.

Director: But you don't like this point?

Physician: Who wants to spend time with their enemies?

Director: Why, someone bent on healing, my friend. If you can heal your enemies, imagine what you can do with others, friends and neutrals alike!

Physician: Yes, but I'm not sure there's much I can do with my enemies.

Director: Why not?

Physician: Because their sickness has deep roots.

Director: What would you call this sickness?

Physician: Moral sickness. And it's very hard to cure.

67

Director: This sickness has roots like some terrible weed?

Physician: Yes, that puts it well.

Director: Then uproot the weed.

Physician: But it's not that simple!

Director: Why not?

Physician: Do you have any idea how traumatic an uprooting is?

Director: We need a more gentle uprooting? Then maybe we should put down a few drops of poison for the roots to drink up, to loosen them up.

Physician: What poison do you have in mind?

Director: What can't this particular type of weed stand?

Physician: Moral health. But don't say that's a poison.

Director: No, let's not say that. In fact, let's forget the whole weedy metaphor. So how will you heal? Will you be an example?

Physician: What enemy would follow my example?

Director: Then what will you do?

Physician: Show the advantages of health.

Director: Ah, a what's-in-it-for-me healing. So what's one of the advantages?

Physician: Having good friends.

Director: Something the unhealthy lack?

Physician: Very much so.

Director: What's the advantage of having good friends?

Physician: There are many advantages.

Director: What's the most important?

Physician: They make you feel proud.

Director: Of them?

Physician: Yes, but also of yourself for having them.

Director: And pride can be healthy?

Physician: Why do you ask?

Director: Because we spoke of boundless pride as problem.

Physician: Of course we're not speaking of boundless pride.

Director: And we're certainly not speaking of arrogance. But that's something your enemies have, isn't it?

Physician: Yes, in abundance.

Director: Can you help turn their arrogance into proper pride?

Physician: Maybe. But that's a very difficult thing.

Director: Where would you start?

Physician: With the desire.

Director: The desire?

Physician: The desire to learn true pride. If they lack that, there's nothing I can do.

Director: So let's say they want to learn. What do you teach?

Physician: I teach them to see themselves for who they are.

Director: How?

Physician: Through judicious use of praise and blame.

Director: I see a challenge here.

Physician: Ha! There are many challenges here. Which do you have in mind?

Director: The sick might think the praise is insincere.

Physician: Why would they think that?

Director: Because they're very sensitive to this.

Physician: Why are they so sensitive?

Director: Because they're open to the cure. And in their openness they want the pure cure and nothing less.

Physician: So what's the pure cure? Honest praise?

Director: Honest praise.

Physician: But why wouldn't the praise be honest?

Director: Because the praise giver doesn't want to discourage the sick.

Physician: So the praise giver inflates the praise?

Director: Right. And there's more. The blame, too, must be honest.

Physician: The sick will know if you're holding back?

Director: They will. Assuming, of course, these sick are ones worth healing.

Physician: Then how do we give honest blame?

Director: By giving a full and accurate description — of the effect of the sick ones' ways.

68

Physician: What's an effect of the sick ones' ways on others?

Director: Others? Can't we think of many? Why don't you tell me one you're particularly concerned with?

Physician: Injuring someone's confidence.

Director: What's an example?

Physician: You might have a fledgling belief that you can be a great leader some day...

Director: ...and an arrogant one comes along and undermines this belief.

Physician: Yes.

Director: But what if you really have no chance of becoming a leader? Is it bad to set you straight?

Physician: Why wouldn't you have a chance? Doesn't everyone have a chance, even if only for a humble leadership role?

Director: But what if it's clear you're not willing to do what it takes? Leadership does take something, doesn't it?

Physician: Of course it does.

Director: So in that case, the bad one, in discouraging your belief, the belief that you can lead without doing what it takes — did something good?

Physician: I don't like to say it.

Director: Would it be better if a good one did this good?

Physician: Yes, because a good one would do more.

Director: What more?

Physician: Encourage you to do what needs to be done.

Director: But what if you simply refuse to do it?

Physician: Then the good one will suggest something else.

Director: Something that can give you confidence?

Physician: Yes, you must reject the old, false confidence — and take up the new.

Director: What if you only take up the new half way?

Physician: You mean, you hold secret hopes for the old?

Director: Don't you think that happens?

Physician: I do. And I think it's a shame.

Director: Why?

Physician: Because you'll never fully have your new and true confidence if you don't cut ties with the old.

Director: Cutting ties can be very hard.

Physician: You don't have to tell me.

Director: When you cut ties, do you change your reality?

Physician: I think that's a very good point. You absolutely do.

Director: So we can all change reality, at least to some degree?

Physician: Yes, but I don't like what you're suggesting.

Director: Oh? Why not?

Physician: Not all of us need to cut ties in order to change.

Director: That's true. And we should note that we're not saying all change is good.

Physician: We're certainly not. There's plenty of good that hasn't changed in a thousand years.

Director: Then is this true? The healthy know what needs to change and what should remain the same.

Physician: Yes, the sick don't know these things.

Director: And is that how you minister to them? You teach them these things?

Physician: Of course. And they need to know there are two types of change. Change in yourself and change in the world.

Director: But doesn't that amount to much the same thing? Didn't someone once say, 'Change yourself and change the world'?

Physician: There's truth in that saying. So we'll tell the sick to change themselves.

Director: How do we get them to change?

Physician: As we said. We start by showing them the advantages of being well.

Director: But what if they're disgusted by those advantages?

Physician: Then they'll never be well. But why would they be disgusted?

Director: Oh, who can say with the sick? Something rubs them the wrong way, and there you have it — disgust.

Physician: Then they need to learn not to be disgusted.

Director: Yes, but learning that is hard.

Physician: And that's how we know it's good.

69

Director: Tell me, Physician. Do you think learning is always healthy?

Physician: Of course I do. Don't you?

Director: I don't know. Have you ever learned something that made you sick?

Physician: What, you mean, for instance, learning about the cruelties some people inflict on animals? Yes, I've learned some things that have made me sick.

Director: Did your sickness lead to health?

Physician: Yes, but I had to take action first.

Director: What action?

Physician: I got involved in a society to protect animals.

Director: And that made you feel good, made you well?

Physician: Yes, it did.

Director: Tell me. Those who torment animals, do they have a conscience?

Physician: Absolutely not. And they're very, very sick.

Director: Are they less sick if they do in fact have consciences, but their consciences are asleep?

Physician: If you're not actively listening to conscience, what difference does it make?

Director: Can we wake their consciences up?

Physician: I think we can.

Director: What needs to be done?

Physician: We have to strike fear in their hearts.

Director: Fear? Are you sure?

Physician: What other way to rouse a slumbering conscience?

Director: So let's suppose we've struck this fear. What happens then?

Physician: They might be motivated to change their lives.

Director: But it's different when someone has no conscience, not even one that sleeps?

Physician: Very different.

Director: What's to be done with them?

Physician: They have to learn right from wrong from scratch.

Director: What would motivate them to do so?

Physician: Who can say? But I do think it happens from time to time.

Director: So how do they learn?

Physician: Someone would have to teach them.

Director: And how did this 'someone' come to learn what's right or wrong?

Physician: Someone in turn taught them.

Director: And who taught this other someone?

Physician: Oh, you're being impossible.

Director: Am I? Didn't someone ultimately have to learn these things first hand, learn them on their own?

Physician: And who do you think that was?

Director: Maybe someone bad.

70

Physician: Why someone bad?

Director: Because what else would you call someone who doesn't know right from wrong?

Physician: Do you think the first humans didn't know right from wrong?

Director: Well, take one of the creation stories. Humans were in paradise. But what did they know?

Physician: I know what they didn't know. They didn't know good and evil until they tasted the fruit.

Director: Yes.

Physician: But that doesn't mean they were bad before they learned.

Director: What were they, then?

Physician: I don't know. Perfect?

Director: Could be. But weren't they bad when they learned? After all, they were told not to eat the apple. They disobeyed.

Physician: That's true. So what are we saying? Learning makes you bad?

Director: I don't know if I'd say that. Maybe the point is that learning certain things makes you bad?

Physician: Good and evil? But what's wrong with learning good?

Director: It seems that knowledge of evil accompanies knowledge of good.

Physician: So there's no learning just one?

Director: At least not at first. But what about health?

Physician: What about it?

Director: Weren't they in perfect health before the fall?

Physician: True, so far as we know.

Director: So they were healthier when they didn't know. How does that sound to you?

Physician: It doesn't sound good.

Director: Why?

Physician: What does it say about knowledge? That it harms? I have a problem with that. Knowledge heals.

Director: But were the first humans in their original state in need of being healed?

Physician: Maybe not. But when they knew, when they fell — there was sickness.

Director: Was the sickness the result of knowledge? Or was it the result of being cast out of paradise?

Physician: What difference does it make? They were cast out because of their knowledge, the knowledge that was prohibited. I don't like the whole thing.

Director: Then let's move on. What do we get from our knowledge of good and evil, however found?

Physician: We know what to do and what not to do.

Director: But does everyone do and avoid as they should?

Physician: Of course not.

Director: Why would someone not do good?

Physician: I don't know.

Director: And why would someone do evil?

Physician: Again, I don't know.

Director: But you know why someone does good and avoids evil?

Physician: Of course. It's for the sake of health.

Director: And if someone does the opposite?

Physician: They'll make themselves sick.

Director: So they harm themselves.

Physician: And others, too.

Director: Can we ever harm ourselves and not harm others, too?

Physician: No, and that's a very important point.

Director: So harming ourselves is evil.

Physician: Yes.

Director: Well, now I'm persuaded to tell you, my friend. There was a time when I harmed myself.

Physician: I'm sorry to hear it, Director. But what harm did you do?

Director: I smothered my thoughts.

Physician: You mean you didn't let them see the light of day?

Director: Yes, in a way. I didn't let them be the light of day in my mind.

Physician: What was your cure?

Director: What else but letting them shine?

Physician: Yes, but did you only let them shine for yourself, or did you let them shine for others?

Director: An excellent question. First and foremost, I let them shine for me.

Physician: And then for others as you saw fit?

Director: Just so.

Physician: That only seems healthy to me. And now you do much good!

Director: What good?

Physician: Why, you help! You help others! We have to help others once we've helped ourselves. That's the only way it all makes sense.

71

Director: Now, to be sure, we're talking about mental health.

Physician: Yes, but the same holds for physical health, you know.

Director: We should help others with their physical health once we've helped ourselves?

Physician: Certainly. And do you know what we can do?

Director: I suppose there are many things we can do. But we might focus on helping them train their bodies.

Physician: Yes.

Director: But is it the same for the mind?

Physician: Can we help train the mind? Of course!

Director: How we help train the body seems obvious. But how do we help train the mind?

Physician: We have to help the person get in the habit of thinking good thoughts.

Director: We should all get in that habit?

Physician: Do you have any doubt?

Director: Maybe not so much a doubt as a question. What's a good thought? A thought that helps us when we think it?

Physician: That's a fine definition.

Director: So how about an example?

Physician: You can say to yourself, 'I'm a good person.'

Director: Saying we're good helps us become healthy?

Physician: Yes, just as saying we're bad has the opposite effect.

Director: But is it enough to say you're good, or do you have to believe it?

Physician: You certainly have to believe it.

Director: And is it enough to believe it or do you have to do something about it?

Physician: No doubt you must do something about it, too.

Director: And when we've done something about it, what do we do?

Physician: I don't know.

Director: Don't we gather up the evidence and weigh it, to see where we stand?

Physician: The good in one scale, the bad in the other?

Director: Yes. We weigh our good and bad and then we know what to think of ourselves.

Physician: That makes sense.

Director: If the good outweighs the bad, we think of ourselves as good. And it's healthy for us to think this way.

Physician: It is.

Director: But if the bad outweighs the good, what happens if we think of ourselves as good? Is that healthy?

Physician: Of course not. We're lying to ourselves.

Director: And if we think of ourselves as bad? Healthy?

Physician: Well, I think it's healthier.

Director: Why?

Physician: Because it's always healthy to tell ourselves the truth.

Director: And that's how we train the mind? We tell ourselves truth?

Physician: Don't you agree?

Director: A mind trained to truth is a wonderful thing. But to know the truth, we have to know the false. Or don't you think that's so?

Physician: No, it's certainly so.

Director: How do we know the false?

Physician: It makes us sick.

Director: It makes everyone sick?

Physician: Eventually? Yes.

Director: Even the bad?

Physician: Even the bad. But they're so used to the false, they don't recognize that it's what's making them sick.

Director: And they might be so used to being sick, they don't even know they're sick?

Physician: Well, I don't know about that.

Director: Okay. But those accustomed to truth and health, do they recognize the false right away because of how it makes them feel?

Physician: They do.

Director: Hmm. Now I don't know.

Physician: What don't you know?

Director: What if a new truth comes along and it makes us feel uneasy?

Physician: We have to get used to it.

Director: But what if before we get used to it, we come to think it's false?

Physician: Well, that's a problem.

Director: So what do we do?

Physician: We have to prove to ourselves whether it's true or false.

Director: Do we also have to do that for things we think are true?

Physician: Prove that they're not false? Yes, we do.

Director: So we have to prove everything as true or false, and this is healthy.

Physician: It is healthy.

Director: How do we prove what something is?

Physician: You mean whether it's false or true? We test it over time.

Director: So we have to be patient.

Physician: Very.

Director: But the reward is worth it?

Physician: Health is worth it.

Director: And just to be perfectly clear, there is no health unless we sift the false from the true.

Physician: Of course not.

Director: And this is something people do every day.

Physician: They do it so often that they're not even aware they're doing it.

Director: What's this? How can we do something without being aware we're doing it?

Physician: What do you mean? It happens all the time!

Director: So the test of truth just happens like that all the time?

Physician: Absolutely!

Director: I don't know about this.

Physician: Why not?

Director: Do you agree there are many things that seem to be true but are actually false?

Physician: I agree.

Director: And those false things can slip through our nets? Or does our automatic testing for truth never let anything false go by?

Physician: No, things slip by.

Director: When is something more likely to slip? When we're running on automatic, or when we actively scrutinize things?

Physician: I see your point. It's best to actively scrutinize.

Director: Suppose we live in a world where there are myriad things coming at us all the time. Wouldn't active scrutiny be exhausting?

Physician: We do live in such a world. And yes, it's exhausting.

Director: If there were those who got by completely on automatic, wouldn't they seem best able to keep up with this world?

Physician: They would. They'd make their decisions right away.

Director: And those who take their time and scrutinize — what happens to them?

Physician: They're accused of slowing things down.

Director: Because those on automatic are impatient.

Physician: Exactly so.

Director: And it seems likely they're not very healthy.

Physician: How could they be healthy?

Director: But those of us who scrutinize?

Physician: We're much more healthy, even though it seems we can't keep up.

Director: What can we do about keeping up?

Physician: We can be selective in what we examine.

Director: How?

Physician: We choose the important things. And let the unimportant go.

72

Director: Do we have to train our minds to let things go? Or does that just happen naturally? Do you know what I'm asking?

Physician: I do. I think it varies from person to person. It's in some people's nature to scrutinize everything, no matter how small. But others just let everything slide.

Director: So a different type of training is required for each?

Physician: Yes.

Director: And both can be healthy if properly trained?

Physician: If both learn to focus on the important, and only on the important — yes, both can be healthy if properly trained.

Director: Is this how you'll train your students?

Physician: Give them more than they can handle and expect them to pick out the important? That seems a little cruel.

Director: You'd rather give them only the important?

Physician: Yes, of course.

Director: But then your training doesn't mirror life.

Physician: Well, you do have a point. But do you expect me to give them false things, too?

Director: Of course. They need to learn how to discard the false.

Physician: And challenge those who take the false up?

Director: Naturally.

Physician: But my colleagues will attack me for such training, you know.

Director: Because they know a better way?

Physician: No, they don't.

Director: Then go your own way, and teach your students the skills they need for health.

Physician: You make it sound so easy.

Director: I don't mean to. There's nothing harder than teaching health.

Physician: Not even philosophy?

Director: I'm assuming philosophy will be part of your teaching.

Physician: Ha! You're looking for a teaching job?

Director: Under the right circumstances, maybe. But don't you think philosophy involves the weighing of true and false?

Physician: I'd go so far as to say that's what philosophy is.

Director: If you're right, then you must become a philosopher.

Physician: And my students, too?

Director: Yes, philosophy for one and all.

Physician: For the sake of truth.

Director: For the sake of health.

Physician: But is everyone cut out for philosophy?

Director: That's the thing. You must fail the ones who aren't.

Physician: Oh, but how can I do that? Do you have any idea what kind of pressure I'd face from my peers?

Director: What's their argument? That the truth isn't important?

Physician: Of course they think the truth is important.

Director: Then I don't see what the problem is.

73

Physician: The problem is they think they know the truth about health and don't like philosophers who question.

Director: Do they harbor untruths?

Physician: I'm sure many of them do.

Director: These untruths are treacherous things. You'll have to teach your students how to deal with them.

Physician: How do you think I can do that?

Director: Why, you might openly confront those who deal in untruth. Your students can watch and learn.

Physician: Ha! You just want me to be at war with everyone.

Director: No, I just want you to be at war with important myths.

Physician: Like I said — you want me to be at war with everyone!

Director: Do you really think things are all that bad?

Physician: Maybe not. But even though my peers might not 'deal' in untruth, they still might tell themselves lies.

Director: How do they tell themselves lies?

Physician: Do you agree that every untruth has its signs?

Director: Signs that reveal its nature? I do.

Physician: When we see these signs, don't we often ignore them?

Director: Many people do.

Physician: Do you know why?

Director: Because they want to believe the untrue is true.

Physician: Exactly. So ignoring and believing amounts to a lie. What do you think?

Director: I think you're telling truth. But are we looking for perfect honesty with ourselves?

Physician: We are. And do you know who I think can be so honest?

Director: I don't.

Physician: A philosopher!

Director: Yes, but now I have a question. When someone is honest with themselves, does that honesty always translate into honesty with others?

Physician: Always? No, I don't think so.

Director: Why not?

Physician: Why not? Ha! Who knows all the reasons why a person would lie?

Director: I think I know one of those reasons.

Physician: Oh? What?

Director: Because someone is lying to you.

Physician: Do you think that's a good reason?

Director: I think it depends.

Physician: Can you give an example?

Director: Sure. What if you know one of your students is being dishonest with you?

Physician: I'd consider that all the more reason to be honest with them.

Director: You'd tell them the truth, which is that you see through their lies?

Physician: Absolutely.

Director: But what if they're lying in self-defense?

Physician: Why would they do that?

Director: Because they're afraid to open up.

Physician: But they want to open up, to open up to the truth, to health?

Director: Yes, very badly. But their fear won't let them. So what do you think? Would you be fully honest and call them on their lies?

Physician: I'd be more gentle.

Director: You'd pretend not to see what you see?

Physician: Well, yes, in a way. But I'd try to open them up by giving them truth, some truth about health.

Director: And if they open up? Do you know what to do?

Physician: Of course. But you tell me.

Director: Engage in fair trade, more of your truth for theirs.

Physician: Yes, but I'll have more truth to give.

Director: Are you so sure?

Physician: Why shouldn't I be?

Director: Look at it this way. Won't you find much to be of interest in someone like this?

Physician: Of course.

Director: And when there's much interest, aren't there many truths?

Physician: Certainly. And these are the truths they'll trade for mine?

Director: Yes.

Physician: Then I see what you mean. I should never take more than I give.

Director: Why not?

Physician: Because what would that say about me?

Director: It would say you're willing to learn.

Physician: But what about fair trade?

Director: As you learn you'll start to develop more truths of your own, truths you can share with others.

Physician: Yes, but how do I repay the student who taught me?

Director: You can give them good grades.

74

Physician: But what if they don't do well in class?

Director: You'll have to figure it out. But let's get back to the false.

Physician: What false?

Director: The falsehoods you'll tell your class so they can learn to sift the truth.

Physician: I have a way of feeling better about this.

Director: Oh?

Physician: I'll tell my students ahead of time that I'll be throwing falsehood in.

Director: They'll know what to expect? Is that how it is in life?

Physician: Well, no.

Director: Then why make it easier on them?

Physician: Director, you're being impossible. Students expect they'll get the truth from the professor.

Director: And do they always?

Physician: Of course not.

Director: How can they tell?

Physician: They have to think things through.

Director: And you don't want your students to think things through? You want to hand them things on a platter?

Physician: I'd love to see you try to teach.

Director: I think it might be fun.

Physician: Fun? Teaching is serious work.

Director: I'm sure it can be. Especially if everything you say is true.

Physician: I don't believe anything you've said. I think you're testing me!

Director: Could be, Physician. But do you admit I have a point?

Physician: What point?

Director: That a healthy student must learn to deal with falsehood that comes when it's least expected.

Physician: Yes, that's true. And they can get that experience outside my class.

Director: In the classes of your peers?

Physician: Right.

Director: Hmm. What happens if a professor has good intentions, and they want their students to be as healthy as can be — but the professor sometimes says what's false?

Physician: Unintentionally?

Director: Yes.

Physician: That's the hardest falsehood to guard against. It's treacherous, as you said.

Director: Is it better to have a snake of a professor who deliberately speaks what's false?

Physician: With no warning to the students?

Director: With none, but with extra credit for those who figure it out, and full disclosure later on.

Physician: I don't care about extra credit and full disclosure. The students need to know what's happening as it happens.

Director: Okay. But what about a snake of a professor who always speaks the truth?

Physician: But then why is he or she a snake?

Director: Because some feel this truth comes at just the wrong time.

Physician: It deliberately comes at that time?

Director: Deliberately, yes.

Physician: But what would be the point?

Director: To bring certain conceited people down a notch or two.

Physician: And would they be healthier for it?

Director: Yes.

Physician: But how can you be so sure?

Director: Let me ask you something. Have you seen the caduceus?

Physician: Of course I have. It's the symbol of medicine.

Director: What's striking about the symbol?

Physician: The two intertwined snakes! Ha, ha! I hadn't thought of that. But the true symbol is the rod of Asclepius, the god of healing, with just a single snake.

Director: Well, if we see signs our snake of a professor is acting on behalf of the god...

Physician: ...then we should remember truth heals — and take the snake's timing on trust.

75

Director: What's left to say about health?

Physician: We can always say more about the proper working of the body.

Director: Yes, and I suppose we can also say much more about the proper functioning of the mind.

Physician: Then how do we narrow things down for the time we have left?

Director: The time we have left.... I wonder. How long should a healthy body live?

Physician: You're asking me?

Director: Yes, at what age should we die?

Physician: We should die when we've lived a good and full life.

Director: And how long does that take?

Physician: Who can say?

Director: Is twenty-five a good age?

Physician: No! That's much too young.

Director: How about fifty?

Physician: Well....

Director: What about seven hundred and twenty-seven?

Physician: Ha, ha. That might be a little too old.

Director: Can the life expectancies we calculate help us here?

Physician: How would they?

Director: They might tell us when our good and full lives should come to a close.

Physician: Oh, they don't tell us that.

Director: What do they tell us?

Physician: How long people, on average, will live.

Director: And that's mere life with nothing to do with goodness and fullness, with health?

Physician: Yes.

Director: What part of our health has most to do with goodness and fullness?

Physician: What part? I'll tell you the order of parts from most to least important. Heart, mind, society, body.

Director: So, a healthy heart, in the metaphorical sense, is the key.

Physician: Don't you agree? But why do you say 'metaphorical'?

Director: Because you're not talking about the blood-pumping organ. You're talking about something else. So where is that something else? I take it you're not thinking of it as a literal part of the body.

Physician: No, I'm not.

Director: And I take it you're not thinking of it as a part of society.

Physician: Of course not.

Director: So what does that leave us but mind?

Physician: The heart is part of the mind?

Director: That's what I'm led to think.

Physician: Better to say the heart is all of us, the sum of our parts.

Director: That's fine. So to live a good and full life we need a strong heart.

Physician: Yes.

Director: And when our heart stops beating strongly?

Physician: We're ready to die?

Director: You're not sure?

Physician: There are times in our lives when our strong heart grows weak. That doesn't mean it's time to die. It might again grow strong.

Director: So how do we know when it's time to die?

Physician: We don't.

Director: I don't know, Physician. I think some people know.

Physician: How do they know?

Director: I don't know. They just seem to know.

Physician: I know you're not satisfied with that for an answer.

Director: Maybe they sense things are slowing down in a final sort of way.

Physician: What tells them this is so?

Director: Their mind.

Physician: Yes, but many people at advanced ages have trouble with their minds.

Director: Maybe they're not the ones who know when it's time.

Physician: That hardly seems fair.

Director: We all should know?

Physician: Yes. So what in particular about the mind lets us know?

Director: Its independence.

Physician: And what do you mean by that?

Director: The ability to focus wholly on yourself.

Physician: That's a strange definition.

Director: Do you think it's false?

Physician: I'm not sure. But if we weren't talking about death, I'd say it's selfish.

Director: There's nothing selfish in a bad way in this.

Physician: Being completely self-absorbed isn't selfish?

Director: Oh, we're not talking about being completely self-absorbed. Just because we're able to concentrate on ourselves, that doesn't mean it's all we ever do.

Physician: So independent minds focus on others?

Director: Of course.

Physician: Okay. But what about when we're not at death's door? Should we be independent in your sense then?

Director: How can we know we're not at death's door?

Physician: Well, that's true. But what if some of us need assistance?

Director: Assistance focusing on ourselves? There's nothing wrong with that.

Physician: Do you think you might need some help?

Director: Me? I wouldn't turn it down, if it really helped.

Physician: What do you think it might involve?

Director: Surgery.

Physician: What?

Director: Surgery to implant a device to help me think.

Physician: Ha! You can't be serious! But I'm curious. So tell me. Are you in control of this device?

Director: Yes. And it allows me to make myself independent.

Physician: But only if you really learn to use it, and then you use it well?

Director: Of course.

Physician: But what if the device were monitored and controlled by others?

Director: You mean, they'd ensure I'm independent?

Physician: No, that's not what I mean. I mean, don't you lose your independence that way?

Director: Because of others in my mind?

Physician: Yes!

Director: I suppose it would be a distraction.

Physician: A distraction? Ha! You're joking, right?

Director: I am. But tell me what you think about this. What if the device is programmed to monitor thought, and make healthy adjustments, but without any control by you or anyone else? And you can turn it off or on. Independent?

Physician: Are you asking in earnest?

Director: Yes.

Physician: Of course you're not independent, unless you leave it off.

Director: Why?

Physician: Because we need to be totally free in our minds!

Director: So you'd never join a cult?

Physician: What? Ha, ha. Now you're being ridiculous. Of course I'd never join.

Director: What if you were born into one?

Physician: Well, they would try to program me.

Director: And if they did, would you be independent?

Physician: No, I wouldn't.

Director: You'd have to resist if you wanted your independence?

Physician: I would.

Director: Now, it's one thing to know something is bad and you want to resist. But it's another thing to know where to go from there. Do you agree?

Physician: Certainly.

Director: So is it good to blindly resist? Or should you know where you're going first?

Physician: I'm not sure.

Director: Why not?

Physician: Because if you wait until you know where you're going, it might be too late.

Director: So why not steer by your health?

Physician: You mean, go where you feel healthy?

Director: Yes. What's wrong with that?

Physician: You might not have enough experience to know where health is.

Director: So you might feel sick and think it's health?

Physician: No, that's not what I mean.

Director: What do you mean? Do you think we all know health when we feel it?

Physician: Yes.

Director: So why not follow health and let all else be damned?

Physician: Because.... Because....

Director: Because why?

Physician: Because we have responsibilities!

Director: To whom?

Physician: To the other young ones in the cult.

Director: We can't leave them behind?

Physician: No, we can't. We have to get them out.

Director: But what if they're happy there?

Physician: How could they be?

Director: You might as well ask why there are cults.

Physician: Why do you think there are?

Director: Because they promise happiness, health, and belonging — and some people can't resist.

76

Physician: You know, it's not just cults that do this. Think of the whole advertising industry.

Director: True. So how should we respond to such promises?

Physician: We have to weigh the claims accurately, and see things for what they are.

Director: Do you believe if we all could see through false promises, the world would be a better place?

Physician: I have no doubt about that.

Director: So we should all learn to weigh and judge.

Physician: Yes.

Director: And is it enough to weigh and judge, or do we have to learn to weigh and judge well?

Physician: Of course we have to learn.

Director: Which is worse? Not to weigh and judge, or not to weigh and judge well?

Physician: I'm not sure it makes any difference.

Director: Oh, but I think it does make a difference. When we don't weigh and judge well, we have an opportunity to learn and improve. But if we don't even try....

Physician: I take your point. We'll never learn.

Director: And the more we learn, the more closely we can focus on what brings us happiness, belonging, and health.

Physician: Yes, but when you've practiced as long as I have, you see that people don't always learn when it comes to health.

Director: Why wouldn't they?

Physician: Oh, there are a million reasons. Some are too lazy to learn. Some are blinded by ambition or greed. And some are overwhelmed by sorrow.

Director: What about those who are afraid?

Physician: What do you mean?

Director: They're afraid to pursue their health.

Physician: Give me an example.

Director: Someone does unhealthy things because of pressure from their peers.

Physician: I agree. Peer pressure can lead to fear, which can lead to unhealthy things.

Director: So is it a stretch to say that health requires some courage?

Physician: No, it's not. We've spoken of courage.

Director: Yes, but there's more to say.

Physician: What more?

Director: Doesn't it take courage to listen to our bodies?

Physician: Yes, that's certainly true. And that leads to health.

Director: And doesn't it take courage to listen to our minds?

Physician: Of course. And I think that, too, leads to health. But we seem to be implying something I don't like.

Director: Oh? What's that?

Physician: If health takes all this courage, do the cowardly grow sick?

Director: Do they?

Physician: I can't believe I want to say it, but I think they do.

Director: Then there are two points we have to make right now.

Physician: What are they?

Director: First, we're using 'cowardly' in a very specific sense.

Physician: Yes, we are.

Director: Second, and to be especially clear, we're not saying all the sick are cowardly.

Physician: No, it would be crazy to say that.

Director: Because there are a great many times when illness can't be helped.

Physician: No doubt. And in those cases many are courageous.

Director: Because you have to be brave to stand up to your illness.

Physician: You do.

Director: Does it matter what kind of illness we're talking about?

Physician: No, you can be brave fighting any illness.

Director: Even the common cold?

Physician: Well, you want to make it sound ridiculous. But I think it can take some courage, if only a very little, to fight a cold.

Director: What would take more courage?

Physician: Any disease that threatens your life.

Director: And that's where you must put up a terrible fight, a total fight.

Physician: Yes.

Director: But let's clarify something. What exactly takes courage here?

Physician: What do you mean?

Director: Is it facing the prospect of death? Or is it putting up the fight?

Physician: Both take courage.

Director: But which takes more?

Physician: If I had to say? I'd say it's the latter.

Director: Why?

Physician: Because we all face death. But not all of us have to fight.

77

Director: When else do we need courage?

Physician: When it comes to mental health.

Director: Oh, I thought that was included in what we were saying.

Physician: Then when do you think we need courage?

Director: When it prevents us from being cowards.

Physician: Well, of course.

Director: Tell me, Physician. How many people do you think are courageous?

Physician: In general? Who can say?

Director: Can we say how many are cowardly?

Physician: I think we can safely say most people are in-between.

Director: Neither courageous nor cowardly?

Physician: Right.

Director: And if neither courageous nor cowardly, then performing neither courageous nor cowardly acts?

Physician: True.

Director: So these people neither stand up to nor run away from their fear?

Physician: Precisely.

Director: Then here's what I wonder. Will they bow down to what they fear?

Physician: That's what a coward does.

Director: So if we do the opposite, and never bow down — do we know we're brave?

Physician: We do.

Director: But now I wonder this. Can we still be brave if we bow down on occasion?

Physician: Why would we do that?

Director: Because we're acknowledging someone as equally brave.

Physician: The brave never bow down, even to acknowledge the brave.

Director: Then how do they acknowledge?

Physician: They look the person right in the eye.

Director: And that's it?

Physician: Isn't that enough?

Director: You ask this as if I were brave.

Physician: Of course you're brave!

Director: And so are you?

Physician: Have you ever seen me bow down?

Director: No. But I'm afraid for you, Physician.

Physician: Afraid? What are you talking about?

Director: I think you want to bow down.

Physician: To whom?

Director: Your students.

Physician: Why would I bow down to them?

Director: Because you're taken with their potential.

Physician: What potential?

Director: Potential to be healthy. What else?

Physician: Why would I bow to potential and not to the actual fact?

Director: Because potential allows the imagination play.

Physician: And you think I think they'll be healthier than they will?

Director: That's the danger.

Physician: But why is it a danger?

Director: You'll expect too much of them.

Physician: And if I do?

Director: They'll feel they've let you down.

Physician: And that's no healthy feeling to have. So what should I do?

Director: Expect nothing.

Physician: What? But they'll sense that's how I feel toward them!

Director: If a teacher expected nothing of you, what would you do?

Physician: I'd seek to prove them wrong.

Director: Wrong? You mean they should have formed expectations?

Physician: Of course!

Director: But why?

Physician: Because they saw potential in me!

Director: Then they should have recognized that potential — and expected nothing.

Physician: That's what you think I should do? What would be the point?

Director: Of recognition? Why, you offer encouragement.

Physician: Yes, but why expect nothing?

Director: To keep the pressure off.

Physician: But pressure can be good.

Director: Yes, and your students will have plenty of that — in their own lives, outside your class.

Physician: So it's not my job to put pressure on them?

Director: It's your job to see their potential for what it is. But this isn't easy, you know.

Physician: Why not?

Director: Because we're talking about potential for health.

78

Physician: Why is potential for health especially hard to see?

Director: For many? Here are a couple of possible reasons. One, they've never known health themselves so they can't recognize it for what it is in others. Two, they don't have health themselves so they're blinded by jealousy when they start to see it.

Physician: I think you're right that some are jealous. But I don't believe people don't know health when they see it. We all know health when we see it.

Director: Bodily health, maybe — assuming there's nothing rotten beneath the surface. But what about mental health?

Physician: You don't think we can tell when someone is mentally ill?

Director: Can all of us tell? Sometimes, yes, in severe cases. But what about something like a depression which the person hides?

Physician: If you got to know the person well, you'd know about that.

Director: Is that the key, then? Getting to know the person well?

Physician: Of course. And that's what good doctors do.

Director: How do they get to know their patients well? Through high tech exams?

Physician: No, they talk to them.

Director: Ah, talk, the ancient method. Talk will ferret out illness?

Physician: Yes.

Director: Any sort of illness?

Physician: What illness have you got in mind?

Director: Well, I know there are many sorts of officially recognized illnesses — schizophrenia, bipolar disorder, and so on. But what about something more simple?

Physician: Like what?

Director: Believing something is true that's not.

Physician: Give me an example.

Director: You think I'm terribly handsome, but I'm not. Does that sound healthy to you?

Physician: Ha, ha. I'll say no.

Director: So how much more unhealthy is it when it comes to more important things?

Physician: Such as?

Director: You believe you've never done wrong.

Physician: Everyone has done wrong at one time or another.

Director: We're certain about that?

Physician: Of course! No one is perfect.

Director: So if you talk to a patient who is completely convinced that they've never done wrong...

Physician: ...then I know there's something wrong.

Director: And what's the treatment?

Physician: To gently persuade them they've done wrong, like everyone else.

Director: Is that the essence of mental illness?

Physician: What do you mean?

Director: Thinking you're not like everyone else.

Physician: Well, we're all unique, in a sense.

Director: Yes, in a sense. But what if I tell you I think I'm the only true philosopher there's ever been? All other philosophers before me were wrong. A sign of illness?

Physician: I don't know. What if you're just exaggerating to prove a point?

Director: No, I'm not exaggerating. I really believe it. Ill?

Physician: Yes.

Director: And what's the cure?

Physician: To prove to you you're not all alone, that other philosophers were right in their own way.

Director: So I'm to moderate my claims.

Physician: Yes.

Director: Are all immoderate claims signs of mental illness?

Physician: Truly immoderate?

Director: Yes, crazy immoderate.

Physician: Well, when you say 'crazy'....

Director: How about radically immoderate?

Physician: Yes, all radically immoderate claims, claims believed by the one making them, are signs of mental illness.

Director: Are you sure?

Physician: Do we need to get into a discussion of what the radically immoderate is?

Director: Let's save that for another time. But these beliefs, the radically immoderate beliefs, are they always on the surface?

Physician: The surface of the mind? Sometimes. But sometimes you have to dig to get at them.

Director: Why do you think people would bury these beliefs deep down inside?

Physician: I think at some level they know people will have a negative reaction to them.

Director: So they believe in secret.

Physician: Yes.

Director: And is that what a good doctor does? Get at the secret?

Physician: I think it would take a very good doctor, yes.

Director: And when a secret, immoderate belief is found?

Physician: The doctor must show the patient it's not true.

Director: But what if it's true?

Physician: That's a topic for our discussion of what the radically immoderate is.

Director: Fair enough. But is it dangerous to show the patient the belief isn't true?

Physician: Yes.

Director: Why?

Physician: Because beliefs like this are very powerful. You can't expect someone to let go just like that.

Director: So it's best to be patient when working with these beliefs?

Physician: Very patient.

Director: But what if there's no time?

Physician: Why wouldn't there be time?

Director: Because you have many other patients to see. Because you have business elsewhere. There are many possible reasons.

Physician: If there's no time, I suppose you have to be blunt — but only if you think the person has it in them to let go of the immoderate belief.

Director: How can you tell if they do?

Physician: There will be signs.

Director: Signs that they're wavering?

Physician: Yes.

Director: And that they suspect what they believe is beyond all reason?

Physician: They're starting to suspect that, yes.

Director: So I might doubt that I'm the only true philosopher in the world.

Physician: You might.

Director: And when you tell me I'm not, and I accept it because somehow I know it's true....

Physician: You have to go off on your own and come to terms with what you know.

Director: That sounds like a very hard thing to do.

Physician: I'm not sure there's anything harder.

79

Director: Tell me something, Physician. Can the good ever be false?

Physician: If it's false, it's not good. So the answer is no.

Director: What happens when many people believe something is good that really isn't good?

Physician: Nothing good happens. And maybe some harm is done.

Director: So when, for example, many doctors believed leeches and bleedings were good cures for a host of ills?

Physician: Not much good happened. And maybe some harm was done.

Director: Did they cherish their belief?

Physician: I don't know that I'd say they cherished it.

Director: Can you think of an example of something cherished that proved false?

Physician: Well, I suppose people cherished the idea that earth was at the center of the universe, that everything revolved around it.

Director: That's the best example you can think of?

Physician: You don't think it's good?

Director: I guess it will do. So back in the day, when many cherished this idea, no one was considered crazy if they believed in it. Am I right?

Physician: You're right.

Director: But if someone cherished that belief now?

Physician: Someone from our society? They might be considered a little crazy.

Director: But not mentally ill in the official sense.

Physician: Not in the official sense. Though their belief might be a symptom of a more serious problem.

Director: One calling for a formal medical diagnosis?

Physician: Yes. But you can be ill in a less than formal way, in a milder way.

Director: Can you give an example of a mild mental illness?

Physician: Having poor judgment.

Director: We're speaking of mental illness in a very broad sense.

Physician: Yes.

Director: What's another way of being mentally ill?

Physician: Not thinking straight.

Director: And another?

Physician: Being confused.

Director: I have to tell you, Physician. These 'mild' mental illnesses, they don't sound mild to me. They sound serious.

Physician: There's truth in that. If things get bad enough, a formal diagnosis might result.

Director: But usually there is no formal diagnosis?

Physician: That's right. Many have poor judgment from time to time. But no one says they need treatment for mental illness.

Director: But maybe they do.

Physician: Ha, ha. And who's going to give them this treatment?

Director: We are!

Physician: I knew you'd say that.

Director: Why not? Why can't we diagnose and treat the mentally ill? Can't we talk with people and determine if they're not thinking straight?

Physician: Yes, we can. But then what do we do? Show them how to think straight?

Director: Of course! If someone is confused, we can help them be clear.

Physician: And to do that we have to determine the cause of the confusion?

Director: Yes.

Physician: And then we attempt to remove the cause?

Director: Oh, we can't do that.

Physician: Why not?

Director: The sick one must do that on their own. We can show them the cause, but then it's up to them.

Physician: And what does the sick one need to do to remove the cause?

Director: Develop a habit.

Physician: What are you talking about?

Director: If in our illness we're accustomed to thinking A is Z, for instance, and A isn't Z, A is A — then we need to develop the habit of thinking A is A.

Physician: So you're saying we should learn to see everything as itself, and this will make us well, much as we said before?

Director: Yes.

Physician: And this goes for people, too. We must see them as themselves.

Director: It very much goes for people.

Physician: And every person is unique?

Director: What do you think?

Physician: You're going to think I'm terrible.

Director: Why's that?

Physician: Well, first, let me tell you — everyone is unique. You are A. I am B. Someone else is C. And so on and so on into infinity.

Director: That doesn't seem terrible.

Physician: Right. But when you think about something approaching infinity, what do you think about?

Director: Grains of sand on a beach.

Physician: Yes! Now, if I take up a handful of sand, am I going to count each grain as unique, give each its own name, because they all have different shapes under a microscope? Or am I simply going to say it's all sand.

Director: So people are people? Is that what you're trying to say?

Physician: Yes, everyone is P. And P is P, so to speak.

Director: I think we need to exercise some judgment here.

Physician: How so?

Director: We know everyone is unique?

Physician: Yes.

Director: But some are more unique than others?

Physician: I'm not sure.

Director: Let's just suppose for now it's true and see where it takes us. So if it's true, then don't we have to ask who deserves to be more unique than others, as far as we're concerned?

Physician: 'Deserves'? You're more unique or you're not.

Director: You don't like 'deserves'? Is it better if we say 'ought'?

Physician: You're suggesting there's a moral element here?

Director: Is there?

Physician: I don't know, Director.

Director: Let's look at it this way. Suppose you know a hundred people. Of those hundred, one is your good friend. The others you don't like. Is your good friend unique in this set?

Physician: Certainly.

Director: What distinguishes your friend?

Physician: The things we have in common.

Director: The sports you like, the shows you watch, the music that moves you?

Physician: You can be friends without those things.

Director: What do you have in common, then?

Physician: Things of the intellect.

Director: Books?

Physician: Sure, books. But other things, too.

Director: What other things?

Physician: Values.

Director: Values aren't moral?

Physician: Well....

Director: I wonder why you're resisting here.

Physician: Because the true reason we count someone or something as unique, or more unique, is because they're our own.

Director: Ah. How about an example?

Physician: My dog is unique from all the other dogs in the world because he's mine.

Director: And your friend is unique from all the other people in the world because he or she is yours?

Physician: Exactly.

Director: And you're unique...

Physician: ...because I'm my own. Because I'm me.

80

Director: What does having your own have to do with health?

Physician: You can't be healthy unless you have your own.

Director: Why not?

Physician: Because your own reinforces your me.

Director: And the me is the core of health?

Physician: What else if not the me?

Director: Then is that the goal in life? To gather as much of your own as you can, so your me is as strong as it can be?

Physician: I'm tempted to say yes. But your own is qualitative, not quantitative.

Director: So one good friend is worth ninety-nine not-so-good friends?

Physician: Yes.

Director: How do you know if a person is your own?

Physician: You just know.

Director: Is it something you feel?

Physician: Yes. You feel it very strongly.

Director: Is this feeling like love?

Physician: This feeling is love.

Director: We love our own.

Physician: We do.

Director: But do we all properly value our own?

Physician: No, I don't think we do.

Director: How can we tell if someone properly values their own?

Physician: By the way they treat you.

Director: How will they treat you?

Physician: They'll try to see you for who you are.

Director: So they can judge if you belong together?

Physician: Yes.

Director: What's the deciding factor in this?

Physician: Mutual understanding.

Director: But didn't we say you can have that with an enemy?

Physician: Yes, but you don't belong together with an enemy. You belong together with a friend.

Director: So we have belonging and understanding with our own.

Physician: Right.

Director: But tell me. Can we understand others? Or do we only understand enemies and our own?

Physician: Of course we can understand others.

Director: Do we need to understand others, or are enemies and our own enough?

Physician: I think it depends on the person.

Director: There's a type of person who wants to understand more?

Physician: You know there is.

Director: Are there many or few of this type?

Physician: In my experience, there are few.

Director: Now, I'm going to ask you a question that may seem strange. When you want to understand, it means you don't understand. Yes?

Physician: Yes.

Director: So people who understand go from not understanding to understanding?

Physician: Of course.

Director: Can they go from understanding to not understanding?

Physician: Well, they might think they understand and then discover they don't.

Director: That's true. But can they go from true understanding to not understanding?

Physician: No. Once you understand you always understand.

81

Director: Do you think it's heaven to be completely understood by a friend?

Physician: I think it's the definition of heaven.

Director: I thought you'd say pure health was the definition of heaven.

Physician: Let's say being completely understood is a part of pure health.

Director: And everyone wants pure health?

Physician: Who wouldn't?

Director: Indeed. But part of pure health is mental health.

Physician: Of course.

Director: And part of pure sickness is mental sickness.

Physician: That follows.

Director: Is pure sickness the definition of hell?

Physician: I'm sure it is.

Director: If we want to avoid pure sickness, what can we do?

Physician: As far as mental health goes? I don't know.

Director: What's in our control when it comes to mental health?

Physician: Thinking.

Director: And?

Physician: Acting on what we think.

Director: Because thinking isn't enough.

Physician: Of course not.

Director: You know, some would say we can't help but act on what we think.

Physician: It's inevitable?

Director: Yes. So if that's true, what happens if we succeed in thinking things through?

Physician: We'll do what must be done.

Director: And when we do?

Physician: You want to know if we'll be in heaven?

Director: Will we?

Physician: Sure.

Director: And so we're done.

Physician: Done?

Director: With thought.

Physician: Are we ever done with that?

Director: But what are you saying? We can never set down the burden?

Physician: Oh, you're just teasing again. You don't think thought is a burden.

Director: How do I think of it?

Physician: I'll tell you how I do. Thought is a tool.

Director: A tool used for what?

Physician: For happiness and health.

Director: But what about knowledge?

Physician: Knowledge, too, is a tool.

Director: Used for happiness and health?

Physician: Of course. What other end could there be?

Director: Satisfaction.

Physician: But satisfaction goes hand in hand with health and happiness.

Director: That's not always true.

Physician: What, you think you can be unhealthy and unhappy and still feel satisfaction?

Director: I do.

Physician: Maybe fleetingly.

Director: Then tell me, Physician. Do you think satisfaction is a deep feeling?

Physician: Yes, I do.

Director: So you're of the view that the deep can be fleeting?

Physician: Well, I'm not so sure about that.

Director: Why not?

Physician: The fleeting is usually on the surface.

Director: And the lasting is usually in the depths?

Physician: Yes.

Director: Hmm. If we stir the surface, can the surface still be itself?

Physician: Of course. The surface is stirred all the time and it remains the same.

Director: And how about the depths?

Physician: The depths would need time to settle back down before we could call them the same.

Director: Is it easy to stir the depths?

Physician: No, it's not very easy at all.

Director: So if you wanted things to be undisturbed, you'd place them there?

Physician: Yes. But where are you going with this?

Director: What kind of things do people place in the depths?

Physician: Healthy people? Precious memories and truths.

Director: What happens if we stir and disturb these things?

Physician: I suppose they might rise to the surface.

Director: And we don't want that?

Physician: Of course we don't.

Director: Why?

Physician: Because we want to keep them in sight!

Director: How would we lose sight?

Physician: Oh, Director. We're stretching the metaphor too far.

Director: Maybe, but let's stretch it just a little bit more. Is it the chop of the waves on the surface you fear?

Physician: Yes, the waves might carry off or smash what we hold dear.

Director: But not if our precious things rise above and fly up into the wind.

Physician: Ha, ha. Now the metaphor is getting a little crazy.

Director: True, but wouldn't you love to watch them soar?

Physician: Would I? I don't know. We'd have to explore more of what this metaphor means, which I'm not inclined to do right now. But I can tell you one thing I'm sure I'd love.

Director: What?

Physician: To bring my treasured things safely again to the deep.

82

Director: We're almost back at the trailhead.

Physician: Good. I have to admit I'm getting a little tired.

Director: Tired of the hike, or tired of the talk?

Physician: Ha, ha. I never tire of the talk with you.

Director: Why is that?

Physician: Because it's good, healthy talk.

Director: What makes it so?

Physician: We speak freely with one another.

Director: And what happens when two people speak freely?

Physician: They either argue or they agree.

Director: What makes argument healthy?

Physician: If it's friendly argument? There's a good chance you'll learn something new.

Director: And what makes agreement healthy?

Physician: It's the grounds for friendship. But there's a qualification here. It has to be agreement on something true.

Director: Why would anyone not agree on the true?

Physician: Because they don't know the truth.

Director: But doesn't it happen another way, too?

Physician: What way?

Director: One person believes the untrue, but the other doesn't.

Physician: And the other agrees?

Director: Yes.

Physician: Why would they do that?

Director: Maybe they don't want to make waves.

Physician: That's very unhealthy.

Director: We should splash around instead?

Physician: Not splash around, but don't let yourself agree to the false.

Director: And if the other forces the issue?

Physician: All the more reason to resist.

Director: Does it take strength to resist?

Physician: Of course it does.

Director: And if we make a habit of resisting like this, we'll build our strength, and if our strength, our health?

Physician: Absolutely.

Director: But we need to be tactful in our resistance?

Physician: That's best, yes.

Director: So tactful that we make no waves?

Physician: Oh, you can be tactful and still make waves.

Director: Just not tidal waves?

Physician: Ha, ha. Yes.

Director: So you'd never dispense with tact?

Physician: When it's a question of tact or truth, I always choose truth.

Director: And you're healthier for it?

Physician: Yes.

Director: Is there ever a time when truth can be unhealthy?

Physician: For you or the one you tell it to?

Director: Either.

Physician: For you, when you know and speak truth, it's always healthy. And I guess I have to say it's always healthy for the one you speak it to, too.

Director: And the false is always unhealthy?

Physician: It is.

Director: Then how simple all this seems.

Physician: Ha, ha! We could have done without our conversation!

Director: Why do you think we had to have our conversation? Why didn't we just say, 'Truth brings health, and falsehood brings sickness' — and leave it at that?

Physician: Because things are complicated.

Director: What do you mean?

Physician: Our truths aren't always accepted.

Director: I see. But is there any other reason?

Physician: Well, there might be a clash.

Director: A clash of truths?

Physician: I was thinking of a clash of desires.

Director: Ah. If we both want something and only one of us can have it, we'll likely collide. But what does that have to do with falsehood and truth?

Physician: The rivals will be tempted to lie.

Director: Why?

Physician: To gain an advantage.

Director: And if they succeed, they forget all about whatever lies they told, laugh, and say they've won?

Physician: Yes.

Director: And that's their truth, that they've won?

Physician: That's a funny way to put it, but yes — that's their truth.

Director: It's a strange truth, if you ask me.

Physician: Can you say more?

Director: It's a compound truth.

Physician: In what way?

Director: There's the truth of winning, the truth that you were 'best'. But there's also the truth concerning your desire and satisfaction.

Physician: What does that mean?

Director: The truth is that you want to win, you desire to win. And when you win, what becomes clear is the final truth, the amount of satisfaction you have.

Physician: So let's be clear. There are three truths. The truth of the desire. The truth of the victory. And the truth of the satisfaction.

Director: Yes. Which of the three, if any, brings health?

Physician: I guess it would have to be the satisfaction.

Director: The other two don't count?

Physician: In the end? They lead to the third.

Director: But, often enough, the winner isn't content, fulfilled.

Physician: Maybe there was a problem with the desire.

Director: You mean, the winner didn't really want what they thought they wanted?

Physician: Yes. Don't you think that happens?

Director: I do. And when that happens to someone who wins, what winner wants to reveal that truth?

Physician: Exactly.

Director: So the truth is obscured?

Physician: Yes, and the only thing we can't obscure is the victory itself.

Director: And that's good, isn't it?

Physician: Why do you say that?

Director: Because we want to be known as winners. And everyone will know we've won.

Physician: You're being ironic but truthful. Many would rather win than be satisfied.

Director: Tell me. Is it always good both to win and be satisfied?

Physician: Of course.

Director: Even with, for example, certain candidates for office?

Physician: Why wouldn't it be good with them?

Director: Because of the reasons for their desire.

Physician: What reasons?

Director: Well, they might want office because it will make them feel important. And they might want office because it will let them manipulate others. And, finally, they might want it because it will allow them to take revenge.

Physician: That would be quite a candidate! But if those are the reasons, then it's in their interest not to win.

Director: Because those are bad, unhealthy reasons?

Physician: No doubt. Bad and unhealthy for the candidate. And bad and unhealthy for the electorate, too.

83

Director: Well, here we are. Back at the cars.

Physician: I enjoyed our hike! Thanks for bringing me along.

Director: I enjoyed the company. So did any of our talk do any good?

Physician: What do you mean?

Director: For your new teaching job!

Physician: It definitely did!

Director: What will you do if you come across unhealthy 'candidates' in your class?

Physician: I'll take them aside and ask them their reasons.

Director: Why they want what they want?

Physician: Yes.

Director: And if they lie?

Physician: I'll call them out.

Director: You'll say, 'Listen, you, I know you're lying and what you really want is to do something bad'?

Physician: Ha, ha. It's not quite that simple, but something along those lines.

Director: But before you can do that, it will take time to get to know them, won't it?

Physician: Yes, but I'm willing to spend that time.

Director: But are they willing to spend it with you?

Physician: Well, that's the problem.

Director: And it's an even bigger problem if they feel you're on the hunt for their truth.

Physician: I suppose that's true.

Director: Won't they try to put you off?

Physician: I'm not so easily put off.

Director: But sitting the chair of health, won't you be limited? I mean, what will you do? Jump up and chase them across campus?

Physician: You have a point. There's only so much I can do.

Director: And would you do this if you could?

Physician: What?

Director: Ruin the chances of those who have unhealthy desires.

Physician: Well....

Director: What would you do with them?

Physician: Teach them health.

Director: And hope they'll no longer, for instance, manipulate others?

Physician: Not hope — know they'll no longer manipulate others.

Director: And you can know this because you've taught them something better than that?

Physician: Yes.

Director: And you'll teach this 'something better' to the healthy students, too?

Physician: The something better is health. And the answer is yes.

Director: But the healthy students, they'll have less to learn?

Physician: No, we always have more to learn.

Director: Then it seems you'll always have work.

Physician: Yes, I'm fortunate in that. But what about you?

Director: Are you worried philosophy will run out of things to do?

Physician: Ha, ha. No, I wonder if you'll go on studying health.

Director: Physician, can any of us go on without studying health?

Physician: And be healthy? No.

Director: Then you have your answer. But I'll tell you this.

Physician: What?

Director: I think today we've stoked the fire.

Physician: The fire of lifelong learning?

Director: What else? I feel the fire in me. Do you feel the fire in you?

Physician: I do.

Director: And won't you try to light the fire in your students?

Physician: I certainly will.

Director: Well, I wish you luck. But if you have any trouble you can always call me.

Physician: Oh? And what would you bring to help with the flame?

Director: Kindling dried by reason.

Physician: Wonderful! And what about the sparks to set it ablaze?

Director: We could knock together two stones.

Physician: But what does 'stone' stand for?

Director: Those impervious to reason.

Physician: Ha, ha! I'd rather knock them together than have them knock into me!

Director: Yes, and the beauty of the knocking is that it's for a good cause.

Physician: Kindling, sparks, fire. But you know, Director, if we keep our own flames lit, we can just light one flame from another.

Director: That's true, my friend. But it's usually good to have a fallback plan. Because who knows? A terrible wind might come and blow out all our flames.

Physician: Then my students must learn how to make fire. But do you think that's something for an introductory course or for one more advanced?

Director: Fire making? I think you should teach it whenever there's opportunity, in whatever level course. I don't think we should squander our chances here.

Physician: Agreed. But maybe you can come in and help me from time to time?

Director: Of course. Fire making is a basic philosophical skill. I have some experience in this.

Physician: Good! Then you'll come. And when you do, maybe you can check in on me and my health.

Director: I will. But what about me? What do I get out of this?

Physician: Why, you get yet another check-up from me!

Director: Good! I was wondering how I would monitor my health once you were gone.

Physician: Well, now you don't have to worry. But you might get something else, you know.

Director: What might I get?

Physician: The finest pleasure there is.

Director: How can I resist? But what is this pleasure?

Physician: Oh, you know what it is! Every true teacher knows!

Director: Then, teacher, it's only fitting for you to tell me.

Physician: The finest pleasure in the world is seeing the dawn of understanding in your students' eyes.

Director: Then I'll have to settle for second best.

Physician: What are you talking about?

Director: They're your students, Physician. I'll just be a guest. But be sure to call me when it's darkest, which they say is right before dawn. And I'll be there.

Printed in the United States
By Bookmasters